RHEUMATOLOGY

D. R. SWINSON
M.B., B.S., M.R.C.P.

And

W. R. SWINBURN
M.B., M.R.C.P.

Consultant Rheumatologists, Wrightington Hospital, Lancashire

HODDER AND STOUGHTON
LONDON SYDNEY AUCKLAND TORONTO

MODERN NURSING SERIES

General Editors
A. J. HARDING RAINS M.S., F.R.C.S.
Professor of Surgery, Charing Cross Hospital Medical School
Honorary Consultant Surgeon, Charing Cross Hospital
MISS VALERIE HUNT S.R.N., S.C.M., R.N.T.
District Nursing Officer, Avon Health Authority (Teaching)

This Series caters for the needs of a wide range of nursing, medical and ancillary professions. A complete list of titles is available from the Publishers.

British Library Cataloguing in Publication Data
Swinson, D. R.
  Rheumatology. – (Modern nursing series).
  1. Rheumatism
  I. Title II. Swinburn, W. R. III. Series
  616.7'2'0024613   RC927

  ISBN 0 340 22357 X Boards
  ISBN 0 340 22356 1 Unibook Pbk

First printed 1980
Copyright © 1980 D. R. Swinson and W. R. Swinburn

Printed in Great Britain for
Hodder and Stoughton Educational,
a division of Hodder and Stoughton Ltd.,
Mill Road, Dunton Green, Sevenoaks, Kent by
Richard Clay (The Chaucer Press), Ltd.,
Bungay, Suffolk.

Editors' Foreword

The scope of this series has increased since it was first established, and it now serves a wide range of medical, nursing and ancillary professions, in line with the present trend towards the belief that all who care for patients in a clinical context have an increasing amount in common.

The texts are carefully prepared and organized so that they may be readily kept up to date as the rapid developments of medical science demand. The series already includes many popular books on various aspects of medical and nursing care, and reflects the increased emphasis on community care.

The increasing specialization in the medical profession is fully appreciated and the books are often written by physicians or surgeons in conjunction with specialist nurses. For this reason, they will not only cover the syllabus of training of the General Nursing Council, but will be designed to meet the needs of those undertaking training controlled by the Joint Board of Clinical Studies set up in 1970.

Preface

Although this book has been written mainly for nurses we hope that those in other professions working with arthritic patients may find part or all of the book useful.

Wrightington Hospital 1979   D. R. Swinson
                                                    W. R. Swinburn

Contents

Introduction

Fossil skeletons of apeman who lived 2 000 000 years ago show evidence of osteoarthrosis, as do the remains of Java man who lived 500 000 years ago. Egyptian mummies dating from 8000 BC show similar changes. Yet the first Chair in rheumatology in Great Britain was only established in 1953 at Manchester University. Since then there has been a rapid expansion in the speciality. The specialist in rheumatology deals with the medical aspects of diseases of joints and muscles. His training is that of a physician and not a surgeon. There is now in Great Britain one professional society (The Heberden Society) devoted solely to work in the field of rheumatology. Another deals with the wider field of rheumatology and rehabilitation (British Association for Rheumatology and Rehabilitation). Similar professional societies exist in most other countries of Europe and together with the British societies form the European League Against Rheumatism. The European League is itself part of the World League Against Rheumatism.

There are two voluntary organizations. The Arthritis and Rheumatism Council (ARC) functions mainly to raise funds for research, although it does supply the very useful booklets available for patients with arthritic conditions and also supports the publication of one of the specialist journals. The British Rheumatism Association (BRA) works at a more practical level in providing help for individual patients.

In Great Britain, in general practice, 12% of all complaints are due to the rheumatic diseases and in 1969 37 million days were lost from work because of these complaints. Of people with severe, chronic disability, arthritis is responsible in 11% of males and 18% of females.

The fact that arthritic diseases are often chronic and frequently lead to disability demands a different approach in treatment from the so-called acute medical and surgical conditions. For example, in pneumonia or acute appendicitis, relatively little cooperation is needed from the patient and the issue, cure or death is usually quickly decided and permanent disability is rare. In rheumatoid arthritis, however, the patient's cooperation is all important. When the diagnosis is made the patient's whole life style is threatened. A man faces the prospect of possibly long periods off work due to exacerbations of the disease and often inability to retain his present job, with subsequent loss of earnings and a lower standard of living. He may be confined to the house and his wife forced to become the bread-winner. Children may suffer from the altered parental relationships and shortage of money. All these social circumstances of his disease are accompanied by painful joints and uncertainty as to the eventual degree of disability. Women suffer similar uncertainties and have particular difficulties with looking after their children and home. They are perhaps more conscious than men of the deformities that occur and their altered physical appearance.

The rheumatologist, therefore, cannot confine himself to the tra-ditional role of the hospital specialist but must also concern himself with the consequences for his patient of deformity and disability; he must consider his patient's life style and social circumstances and should understand and know when to use the special services of the nurse, physiotherapist, occupational therapist and social worker. He must be aware of the special problems that patients experience when their stay in hospital may last several months.

The use and coordination of various remedial staff leads to the idea of the team approach to chronic diseases. At times in his illness the patient may need medical or surgical advice but later his main need may be help from the community services including those with special skills in nursing or social work. It is important that the different members of the team understand not only their own role in management of each particular patient but also the role and import-ance of their fellow members. This complex relationship with its need for mutual confidence between members of the team needs to grow gradually and such teams cannot be assembled on an ad hoc basis for an occasional patient. It is for this reason, amongst others, that these diseases are often treated in special units, sometimes sep-arated from the acute hospital.

The purpose of this book is to explain the medical aspects of the commoner rheumatic diseases, to describe the various treatments that are available, both medical and surgical, and to demonstrate the contribution of each member of the team in the rehabilitation of the patient, not forgetting that an essential member of that team is the patient himself.

We hope also that the object of the book should be to remind the reader that there are no such things as diseases, only diseased people, each of whom is a unique individual needing our sympathy and support in all aspects of his life.

Recommended Further Reading

Annals of the Rheumatic Diseases. Published 6 times a year by the Arthritis and Rheumatism Council.

Journal of Rheumatology and Rehabilitation. Published quarterly by the British Association for Rheumatology and Rehabilitation.

Arthritis and Rheumatism. Published 6 times a year by the American Rheumatism Association.

Reports on Rheumatic Diseases. Issued at intervals by the ARC.

Bulletins on Rheumatic Diseases. Issued at intervals by the American Arthritis Foundation.

An Introduction to Clinical Rheumatology, by M. Mason and H. L. F. Curry (Pitman Medical).

Arthritis and Allied Conditions, by J. L. Hollander and D. J. McCarty (Lea & Febiger).

Clinical Rheumatology, by J. A. Boyle and W. W. Buchanan (Blackwell Scientific Publications).

Copeman's Textbook of the Rheumatic Diseases. Edited by J. T. Scott (Churchill Livingstone Ltd.).

1
Structure and Physiology of Joints

There are three types of joints in the body; fibrous, cartilaginous and synovial. Only the last two need concern us.

Synovial joints

Synovial joints are so called because they are lined with synovium. Most joints of the body are synovial. The typical structure is shown in Fig. 1.1. In its simplest form a synovial joint consists of two bone ends capped with articular cartilage and joined by a fibrous capsule which is contiguous with the periosteum of the bones. The capsule is lined by a thin vascular membrane known as the synovium. This is known as a diarthrodial joint, as two bones articulate.

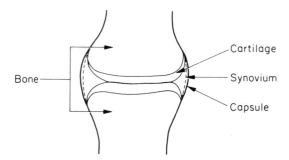

Fig. 1.1 Diagram of typical synovial diarthrodial joint.

Structure and function of articular cartilage. Cartilage is composed of a firm jelly-like substance supported by fibres. Within this substance are scattered the chondrocytes, the cells which produce it and the fibres. The cartilage is designed to absorb shock and to permit movement with little friction within the joint.

The capsule. The capsule is composed of strong interlacing fibres forming a tough protection and support for the joint. Part of the capsule may be thickened and the thickenings are then called ligaments. Ligaments stop excessive movement at a joint. The capsule may also be reinforced by the insertion of muscles and their tendons.

Synovial membrane (synovium). This lines the inside of the joint excepting for the part covered by cartilage. It is formed of a thin layer of cells. These cells produce synovial fluid which in health is thick, clear and sticky and contains hyaluronic acid. It may have a lubricant function. Some of the cells can ingest particles from the synovial fluid, for example, altered blood from a haemorrhage. Synovial membrane also lines other moving structures such as tendon sheaths. This is important when considering the distribution of the effects of diseases such as rheumatoid arthritis which are largely characterized by synovial inflammation.

Nerve supply of synovial joints. The major symptom in arthritis is pain. The nerve endings which produce this pain are mainly located in the joint capsule and surrounding ligaments. The synovial lining of the joint is insensitive. Stimulation of these nerve endings may also cause spasm of muscles acting on the joint and this spasm in itself may be painful.

Cartilaginous joints

Cartilaginous joints are joints where the bone ends are united by cartilage. The most common and most important are the joints between the vertebral bodies in the spine. In these joints, the cartilaginous buffers are called the intervertebral discs (Fig. 1.2). These discs are composed of a tough annulus fibrosus with a jelly-like centre called the nucleus pulposus. This structure is capable of absorbing considerable shock and gives the spine its flexibility. The proximity of nerve roots to this structure is shown in Fig. 1.2 and it is easy to see why disease of a disc may damage the nerves and cause pain in the parts they supply, eg sciatica. When considering the spine, the small apophyseal joints on the posterior part of the neural arch must not be forgotten. These are synovial joints and are particularly liable to various sorts of arthritis.

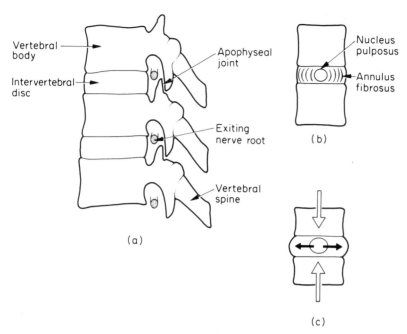

Fig. 1.2 Diagrams to show (a) intervertebral joints, (b) structure of intervertebral disc, and (c) mechanism of discs; vertical forces are translated into lateral forces by nucleus pulposus and absorbed by annulus fibrosus.

Neurocentral joints

Neurocentral joints are small synovial joints found on each side of the intervertebral discs in the cervical spine only (see Fig. 2.10, p. 22).

Further reading

Foundations of Anatomy and Physiology, by J. S. Ross and K. J. W. Wilson (Churchill Livingstone)

2
Osteoarthrosis

Osteoarthrosis (OA) is a disease in which the wearing away of joint cartilage is accompanied by the production of new bone. The new bone appears beneath the worn cartilage and as outgrowths called osteophytes.

Although inflammation may occur in osteoarthrotic joints, it is not a common feature and for this reason the term osteoarthrosis is preferred to osteoarthritis. Sometimes the term degenerative joint disease is used synonymously with osteoarthrosis. Osteoarthrosis is commoner in older people and is sometimes described as 'wear and tear' arthritis. Although there is some truth in this expression, it is important to remember that osteoarthrosis is not an inevitable accompaniment of ageing, nor is it confined to the elderly.

Osteoarthrosis often appears in a joint which has developed abnormally or has been damaged in some way. This is known as secondary osteoarthrosis. When osteoarthrosis arises in a joint where no such preceding disease can be identified it is termed primary osteoarthrosis. When many joints are involved, particularly those of the hand, the condition is known as primary generalized osteoarthrosis (GOA).

A feature peculiar to the spine is the degeneration of the intervertebral discs with subsequent osteophyte production on the edges of the vertebral bodies. This process is called spondylosis and is a similar process to osteoarthrosis occurring elsewhere in the body. In this section the term spondylosis will also include the osteoarthrosis occurring in the apophyseal joints of the spine as well as that occurring in the intervertebral disc joints.

Prevalence

Osteoarthrosis is a common condition. A study in the United Kingdom showed that 20% of the adult population had X-ray evidence of osteoarthrosis. Frequency increased with age so that of those aged 55 to 64, 85% had OA. Much of this radiographic disease is in fact asymptomatic or of only minor clinical significance. However, osteoarthrosis is an important cause of disability in the elderly and provides a major contribution to loss of mobility and therefore loss of independence in these older age groups.

Below the age of 55 the sex incidence is about equal but above this age there is a predominance of women. This is largely accounted for by the high prevalence of osteoarthrosis of the hands in women.

The causes of osteoarthrosis

There are a number of factors important in the causation of osteoarthrosis. The main ones are listed below.

Trauma. Injury to a joint often results in osteoarthrosis. Trauma may be a single event such as a fracture through the joint or may be occupational in origin when repetitive movement results in unnatural wear and osteoarthrosis. A high incidence of osteoarthrosis has been described in miners and in the elbows of people who use vibrating tools and in the hands of cotton workers. Tears of the meniscus of the knee interfere with the distribution of weight within the knee and cause osteoarthrosis some years after the injury. Sports such as football which expose the knee to such an injury are therefore associated with an increased risk of OA.

Other types of arthritis. Inflammatory arthritis such as infection, rheumatoid arthritis or gout may damage a joint and although the original disease may have remitted, the residual damage to the joint results in secondary osteoarthrosis.

Paget's disease of bone may cause a form of secondary osteoarthrosis particularly in the elderly hip.

Congenital and developmental anomalies. These are a relatively common cause of osteoarthrosis. For example, congenital dislocation of the hip (CDH) may vary from complete dislocation of the hips at birth to the presence of shallow acetabuli. This mechanical abnormality produces excessive wear on the joint surfaces and osteoarthrosis supervenes, sometimes while a patient is still in her teens but more usually in middle age. It is likely that much apparent primary osteoarthrosis of the hips in women is in fact secondary to minor degrees of CDH. Perthes' disease is a disease of the epiphysis of the femoral head occurring in children aged 3 to 15. The epiphysis disintegrates causing hip pain, resulting in some cases in a severely deformed femoral head with early secondary osteoarthrosis.

In teenage boys the femoral epiphysis may slip down (adolescent coxa vara) causing a painful hip. This may result in secondary osteoarthrosis with onset of symptoms at any time from the teens to late middle age. Like CDH both these two conditions may occur in mild forms not noticed at the time but eventually resulting in OA.

Metabolic causes. Alkaptonuria is an inherited disease in which an enzyme, homogentisic acid oxidase, is missing. The result is an accumulation of homogentisic acid in cartilage. This gives the cartilage a black colour which gives the disease its alternative name of ochronosis. This results in early degeneration of cartilage and resulting osteoarthrosis. On X-ray calcification is seen in the intervertebral discs and later in the peripheral joints. The disease may be diagnosed clinically by spotting the black pigment in the whites of the eyes and in the ear and cartilage, and by observing the patient's urine which turns black on standing.

This is a rare disease inherited as an autosomal recessive. The importance of this condition is that here we have osteoarthrosis caused by a known enzyme deficiency and marked out easily for us by nature. It is possible that osteoarthrosis in other people may be due to other enzyme defects which do not leave such obvious markers.

Osteoarthrosis may also be associated with chrondrocalsinosis particularly in the elderly and it is possible that the metabolic abnormality is responsible both for the OA and the chondrocalcinosis (Fig. 2.1).

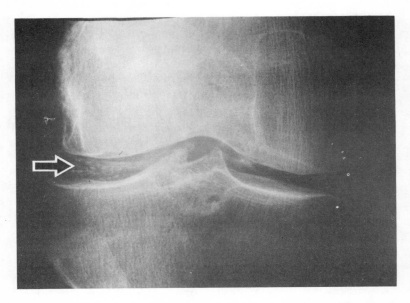

Fig. 2.1 X-ray of knee. Arrow points to calcification in cartilage (chondrocalcinosis).

Recently minute crystals of apatite have been discovered in osteoarthrotic cartilage and it has been suggested that they may induce osteoarthrosis.

Obesity. Obesity is often associated with osteoarthrosis. Although it makes life much more difficult for an osteoarthrotic person, it seems unlikely that obesity is a direct cause of the OA.

Age. The association of osteoarthrosis and age has already been mentioned. There are qualitative differences between cartilage from normal old people and cartilage from old people with osteoarthrosis and it seems unlikely that age as such is a direct cause of osteoarthrosis.

Climate. Although it is a popular idea that rheumatism is associated with dampness, osteoarthrosis occurs in every type of climate but surprisingly enough, it would seem to be less common in Eskimos. However, people in warm climates have less symptoms than those who live in the damp and cold.

Sex and heredity. Osteoarthrosis of the terminal interphalangeal joints of the hand, ie Heberden's nodes, is very much more common in women than men. It appears that there is a strong familial tendency for osteoarthrosis of the hands to be expressed in the female side of the family.

The pathology, clinical features and treatment of peripheral osteoarthrosis will now be discussed. These aspects of spondylosis are referred to later.

Pathology of osteoarthrosis in a diarthrodial joint
(Figs. 2.2 and 2.3)

The first sign is a superficial fissuring of articular cartilage. This is associated with and preceded by chemical changes that take place within the cartilage.

The progression of the condition leads to deeper fissuring of the cartilage with gradual loss of weight-bearing cartilage. Cells which normally are responsible for maintaining the cartilage (chondrocytes) increase in number initially and become more active especially at the base of the fissures. This is probably an attempt to repair the damage. At the same time there is an increased activity of bone beneath the cartilage producing a thickening of the subchondral bone with the production of projections, ie osteophytes.

With continued loss of joint cartilage, cysts form in the bone beneath the cartilage, perhaps caused by pressure forcing fluid through small fractures in the bone.

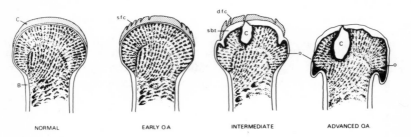

Fig. 2.2 Pathology of osteoarthrosis.
Normal: C, cartilage; B, bone. *Early OA:* s.f.c., superficial fissuring of cartilage. *Intermediate:* d.f.c., deep fissuring of cartilage; s.b.t., subchondral bone thickening; C, cyst; O, a developing osteophyte. *Advanced OA:* shows complete loss of articular cartilage.

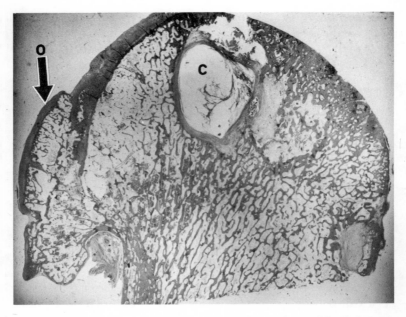

Fig. 2.3 Section through advanced osteoarthrotic femoral head showing loss of cartilage, osteophyte growth (O) and sub-articular cyst (C).

Eventually cartilage is lost completely leaving bare bone which may become polished with friction from use as an articular surface. This is known as eburnation. The cysts that form in the subchondral bone may become large and collapse leading to deformity of the articular surfaces, and subluxation of the joints occurs due to loss of alignment.

Clinical features

Although the symptoms and signs of osteoarthrosis will vary depending on the site of the arthrosis, there are certain features which are characteristic of osteoarthrosis in general.

Pain. The pain from an osteoarthrotic joint is felt characteristically on movement and not at rest. The pain is worse at the end of the day and after exercise. This contrasts with pain from an inflammatory arthritis which is experienced chiefly in the morning and is associated with long periods of morning stiffness.

Sometimes, however, an osteoarthrotic joint may produce an aching pain at rest. This is true particularly of the hip and knee and is thought to be secondary to increased blood flow. Pain may also occur when an osteoarthrotic joint is unconsciously moved in bed at night.

Stiffness. Although stiffness is a feature of inflammatory arthritis, a short spell of morning stiffness lasting less than thirty minutes occurs in osteoarthrosis. Stiffness after prolonged sitting, sometimes termed gelling, also occurs. This phenomenon is unfortunately well recognized in the outpatient waiting room!

Reduction in the range of movement occurs due to muscle spasm which is reversible and due to osteophyte formation which is not reversible.

Clinical features of osteoarthrosis

1. Pain on and after use of joints
2. Mild early morning stiffness and 'gelling'
3. Reduction in range of movement
4. Deformity

Deformity. Deformity due to joint surface destruction and osteophyte formation is common in advanced osteoarthrosis. This is seen particularly in the hands, knees, feet and hip.

Crepitus. This is a crackling sensation produced when an osteoarthrotic joint is moved.

Laboratory and X-ray features

Blood tests in osteoarthrosis reveal a normal ESR and a normal Latex test. An X-ray of an osteoarthrotic joint typically shows loss of joint space because of cartilage destruction, osteophyte formation from the edge of the joint and increased bone density just under the joint space which is called subchondral bone sclerosis. Investigation of the synovial fluid from an osteoarthrotic joint shows a non-inflammatory fluid: ie the fluid is clear, of high viscosity, the number of white cells is less than 1000 and of those less than 25% are polymorphs, and the protein content of the fluid is low. The mucin clot test shows good clot formation.

> Laboratory and X-ray features of osteoarthrosis
>
> 1. Normal ESR and Latex test
> 2. X-rays show loss of joint space, osteophytes and subchondral bone sclerosis
> 3. Non-inflammatory synovial fluid

Local clinical features and treatment

Hands. The joints most frequently involved in osteoarthrosis of the hand are the terminal interphalangeal joints (TIP), the proximal interphalangeal joints (PIP) and the first metacarpal carpal joint (1st MC/C), ie the base of the thumb. The osteophytes produced around the finger joints produce the characteristic deformities which are known as Heberden's nodes at the TIPs and Bouchard's nodes at the PIPs (Fig. 2.4). The condition is commoner in women and the onset often coincides with the menopause. The arthrosis may or may not be painful. Commonly there is pain when the nodes appear and this occasionally may be severe and associated with redness and tenderness. Eventually the pain subsides leaving a stiffer digit and a some-

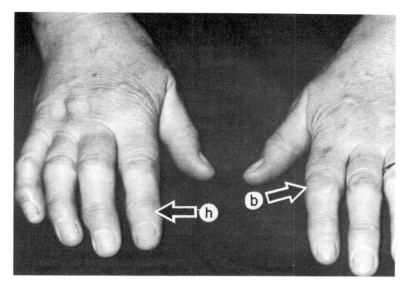

Fig. 2.4 Bony swellings at the TIP joints (h) are Heberden's nodes, similar swellings at the PIP joints (b) are Bouchard's nodes.

what less dextrous but still functioning hand. Osteoarthrosis of the first MC/C joint is again frequently asymptomatic though occasionally very painful. The pain is usually temporary. The squaring of the hand is caused by radial subluxation of the first metacarpal (Fig. 2.5).

Treatment consists of anti-inflammatory analgesic drugs such as aspirin or indomethacin and splinting of the first MC/C joint in a POP splint or in a functional splint to enable otherwise painful hand duties to be performed. Occasionally, local injections of steroid into the first MC/C joint produces relief. Wax baths are also useful in producing temporary relief of pain in some patients. It is very important to reassure patients with osteoarthrosis of the hand that they do not have a crippling condition such as rheumatoid arthritis and often they are quite content if a good prognosis is given. Surgery such as fusion or removal of one of the carpal bones is occasionally used in refractory cases of first MC/C arthrosis.

Osteoarthrosis of the rest of the upper limbs rarely produces a problem. However, conditions such as tennis elbow and peri-articular diseases of the shoulder are common in age groups which suffer from osteoarthrosis elsewhere.

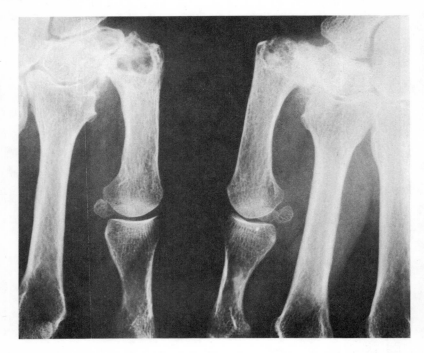

Fig. 2.5   This X-ray shows gross OA of the base of the thumbs (1st MC/C joint) which produces the characteristic squaring of the hand.

Feet. The commonest joint in the foot to develop osteoarthrosis is the big toe joint, ie the first MTP joint. The condition is characterized by much osteophytosis around the MTP joint producing a stiff and painful toe known as hallux rigidus (Fig. 2.6). It is more common in men. Treatment is by adaptations to shoes which prevent or replace the bending of the first MTP joint on walking (Fig. 2.7). If this is ineffective then fusion of the joint or a Keller's operation is indicated.

Hallux valgus is associated with the development of osteoarthrosis of the first MTP joint together with bunion formation (Fig. 2.8). This deformity is commoner in women and is made worse by the wearing of fashionable footwear. Pain in this case is usually due to inflammation of the associated bunion.

The treatment of hallux valgus is surgical and consists essentially of removing the bunion and straightening the first MTP joint with a Keller's operation.

The hind foot may be involved in osteoarthrosis secondary to

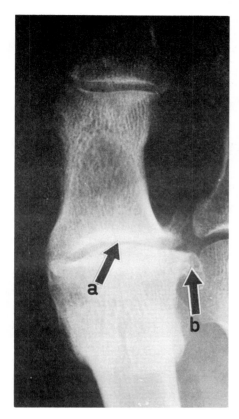

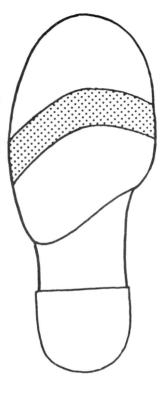

Fig. 2.6 An X-ray to show hallux rigidus: (a) diminished joint space, (b) an osteophyte.

Fig. 2.7 A metatarsal bar across the sole of the shoe diminishes movement at the large toe joint.

rheumatoid arthritis but in primary osteoarthrosis it is very unusual for it to become involved.

Knee. The knee is one of the commoner joints involved in both primary and secondary osteoarthrosis. Being very dependent for stability on tendons and muscles it is more susceptible to trauma than most joints. Pain is felt around the knee and if an effusion is present, at the back of the knee. It is worse on exercise and in severe cases any weight-bearing is very painful and pain may also occur at rest at night. The knees are visibly and palpably enlarged by bony swellings

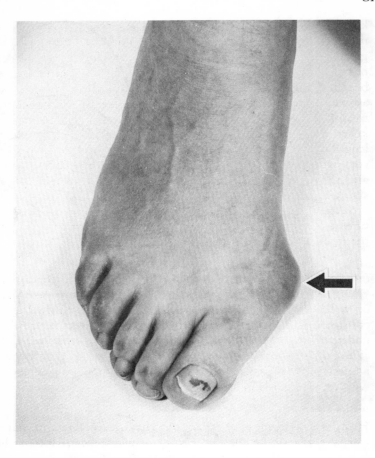

Fig. 2.8   Hallux valgus with bunion (arrowed).

and sometimes enlarged by an effusion. If an effusion is present the pressure within the knee may produce a bulging at the back of the knee, ie a popliteal cyst. This can rupture with results similar to those seen in rheumatoid arthritis. Loss of joint surface and sometimes collapse of the tibial plateau causes instability and valgus (knock knee) or varus (bow leg) deformities. Instability causes more pain due to the stretching of ligaments.

Treatment can be divided into medical and surgical. Medical treatment consists of prescribing analgesics to kill the pain; strengthening quadriceps muscles to their optimum state by exercises to increase knee stability; reducing the amount of weight born on the knees with the use of walking aids; losing weight if obese and if necessary by a short period of bed rest. Local heat may produce a great relief of symptoms particularly in elderly women and occasionally regular physical treatments like this can be of great benefit. Although not a primarily inflammatory disease, joint aspiration and local steroid injection combined with the other treatments above can produce temporary relief. Painful unstable knees are sometimes helped by wearing plastic cylinders or full length calipers. In practice, only a minority of patients seem able to cope with them. Most find them cumbersome and difficult to put on and take off and the cylinders also abrade the skin and tend to slip down.

Surgical operation on the knees may be necessary and consists of tibial osteotomy for moderate cases of osteoarthrotic knees and in the more severe cases some form of arthroplasty can be used.

CHONDROMALACIA PATELLAE. This is a poorly defined condition in young women. The symptoms are knee pain on exercise particularly on walking downstairs. In developed cases quadriceps wasting and effusions occur. Flaking of the cartilage hence chondromalacia on the undersurface of the patella is the chief observable pathology although osteoporosis of the patella is also observed. The prognosis is uncertain. Many fail to recover and this condition probably merges with osteoarthrosis in later life.

Hip. 3.4% of people over the age of 55 have radiological evidence of osteoarthrosis of the hip. Osteoarthrosis may appear without obvious cause or be secondary to such conditions as Legg-Perthés disease, minor forms of congenital dislocation of the hip, slipped epiphysis, aseptic necrosis, inflammatory arthritis or Paget's disease of bone. In the first three conditions symptoms appear in childhood or adolescence and may then subside to reappear in adult life as early osteoarthrosis. Osteoarthrosis secondary to Paget's disease or inflammatory arthritis may be accompanied by pushing inwards of the acetabulum producing a condition known as protrusio acetabulare. Shortening of the affected leg producing a limp may be due to collapse of cysts in the femoral head; apparent shortening is caused by the adduction and flexion deformity of the hip which occurs with advanced osteoarthrosis. Both real and apparent shortening has a profound effect on gait.

The symptoms of osteoarthrosis around the hip are pain, limp and

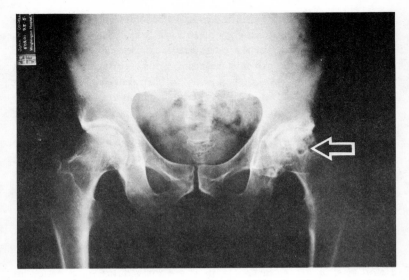

Fig. 2.9 X-ray of pelvis. The left hip is osteoarthrotic. The arrow indicates large cysts in the femoral head.

restriction of movement. The pain is felt around the trochanter, in the groin, thigh and the knee. Backache may be caused by a lordosis secondary to flexion deformity of the affected hip. The pain is initially worse on and after exercise and is usually gradually progressive over months or years. Occasionally pain occurs first when the patient rises from a sitting position. In severe cases pain eventually occurs at rest and at night and this is particularly a feature of hip osteoarthrosis. The gait is affected by pain producing the antalgic gait where the body lurches over the affected hip. Increasing restriction of hip movement by osteophytes eventually produces a shuffling walk. Restriction of hip movement has consequences beyond walking such as difficulty in sitting down, dressing, cutting toe nails, tying shoe laces. In younger women difficulty is experienced in menstrual toilet and sexual intercourse.

Treatment may be by conservative or surgical means. Pain can be ameliorated by anti-inflammatory analgesics. Muscle spasm can be overcome by exercises in a warm pool or sling exercises in the physiotherapy department combined with short wave diathermy. This sort of regimen will produce an increase in pain-free range of movement in most cases. If obese, weight should be lost and for optimum results these conservative measures should be combined

with a period of non weightbearing. A stick used in the hand opposite to the painful hip relieves pressure on that joint when walking.
Intra-articular injections are useful but require performance under
X-ray control. Some patients make a partial recovery but most seem
to progress and need surgery. The most useful form of surgery now
is total hip replacement. This has an acceptable mortality and mor-
bidity even in the elderly and has revolutionized the treatment of
osteoarthrosis of the hip. Alternative procedures still used occasionally particularly in younger patients are intertrochanteric osteotomy
and arthrodesis. Following the former, symptoms are relieved in
about 50% of subjects. The latter produces a painless but stiff joint
and is useful for the young male who might give an arthroplasty an
unacceptable amount of wear.

Spondylosis

Pathology

There are two separate sets of joints in the spine, the intervertebral
disc joints which consist of vertebral bodies separated by the
cartilaginous discs and the apophyseal joints which connect the
vertebral arches posterior to the discs. These latter joints are ordinary
diarthrodial joints and osteoarthrosis affects them in the same way as
described above. Functionally, they are intimately linked with the
disc joints and disc disease here will therefore affect them. Osteoarthrosis in the spine is complicated by the proximity of the affected
joints to the spinal cord and nerve roots. In addition, in the cervical
spine the vertebral arteries are also very close to the affected joints.
Consequently any alteration of anatomy by reason of arthrotic
changes may affect these vital structures.

   The essential event in spondylosis is degeneration of the disc (Fig.
2.11). In disc degeneration the nucleus pulposus loses water and
shrinks. It thereby loses its weight-distributing ability and the body
weight is born by the annulus which is designed to withstand out-
ward pressure from the nucleus but not vertical forces. The annulus
thus damaged is liable to tear particularly if a twisting movement
occurs or if the person lifts with a flexed back. The tear allows
protrusion of part of the nucleus pulposus, the condition known
colloquially as 'slipped disc'. This protrusion is usually backwards or
posterior laterally. The reason for this direction is that the nucleus in
a disc particularly in the lower lumbar spine is situated towards the
back (Fig. 2.12).

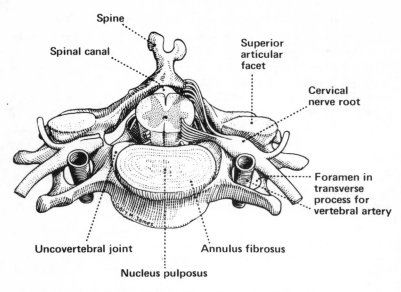

Fig. 2.10 A cervical vertebra, disc and associated structures.
Photograph courtesy of Professor M. I. V. Jayson, W. B. Saunders & Co.
Ltd and Pan Books.

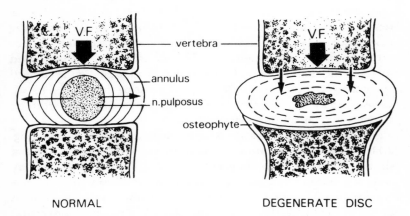

Fig. 2.11 Disc degeneration in spondylosis. VF is vertical force transmitted through spinal column.

In the presence of a normal annulus excess weight bearing may still
produce protrusion of the nucleus but in this case the protrusion is

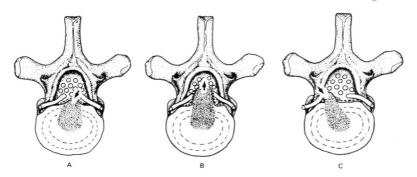

Fig. 2.12 A. Bulging backwards of the nucleus pulposus presses on the very sensitive posterior longitudinal ligament (arrowed) causing low back pain.

B. More severe protrusion through the posterior ligament may compress the spinal cord or cauda equina and produce paraplegia.

C. Posterior lateral protrusion impinges on a nerve root (arrowed) and produces numbness and pain in the distribution of that nerve, eg acute sciatica.

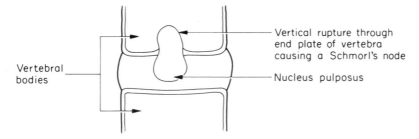

Fig. 2.13 Diagrammatic section through vertebrae to show a Schmorl's node.

central and passes vertically through the end plate of the vertebra producing what is known as a Schmorl's node (Fig. 2.13).

Osteophytes arising from the disc joints and from the apophyseal joints may impinge on nerve roots and the spinal cord particularly in the cervical region (Fig. 2.14). This pressure occurs primarily in the narrow intervertebral foramena. The osteophytic pressure results in scarring of the sensitive and protective dural covering of the nerve roots. Pressure on the spinal cord arises from osteophytes growing from the posterior part of the disc joints.

Osteophytes may also interfere with blood flow through the vertebral arteries which run through the transverse processes of the upper cervical vertebrae.

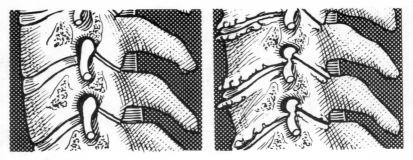

Fig. 2.14 Normal cervical spine on left. On the right, cervical spondylosis is causing osteophyte impingement on exiting nerve roots.
Photograph courtesy of Professor M. I. V. Jayson, W. B. Saunders & Co. Ltd. and Pan Books

Spondylosis is particularly frequent in the lower cervical spine and the lower lumbar spine.

Clinical features of cervical spondylosis

Complaints of neck pain with or without radiation down the arm are very common indeed. Many of these symptoms can be put down to osteoarthrosis of the cervical spine. The symptoms arise either from the joints themselves or neighbouring deep structures such as ligaments and muscles or from nerve root pressure.

Pressure on a particular root results in pain, numbness and paraesthesiae in the area of distribution of that root. There may be associated loss of muscle power and reflexes.

In general involvement of the upper cervical spine causes occipital headaches with forward radiating pain as far as the forehead and eye whilst lower cervical spondylosis causes pain radiating into the shoulders and along the trapezii and down the arms. Pain is made worse by turning the neck and in acute severe cases the head is held in a fixed abnormal position with much muscle spasm (acute wry neck). Pain may be severe and sleeplessness may result. Symptoms may last from days to months and relapses are common. With repeated attacks the range of movement of the neck becomes progressively reduced. The initiating event may be trauma such as a whiplash injury or there may be no definite precipitating cause. The most prominent cause of a whiplash injury is a road traffic accident in which the victim's vehicle is struck sharply from behind and the victim's head is thrown sharply backwards and then forwards.

Similar symptoms to nerve root compression may arise from the arthrotic apophyseal joints as well as other deep tissues. It may be very difficult to distinguish between these symptoms and those arising from nerve root irritation. Very rarely a cervical disc may prolapse backwards and compress the spinal cord resulting in paraplegia. More insidious causes of compression may occur from posterior osteophytes causing a ridge which narrows the spinal canal. This is the syndrome of spinal stenosis.

Vertebrobasilar ischaemia. Osteophytes may cause pressure on the vertebral arteries which are an important means of blood supply to the brain. Interference with blood flow in these vessels causes transient cerebral ischaemia with sensations of dizziness, faintness, weakness and paraesthesiae. Paraesthesiae are characteristically experienced around the mouth. Attacks are usually brought on by moving the neck.

In most cases the symptoms are self limiting although symptoms of numbness and paraesthesiae may persist for a very long time. Relapse is common and may be expected.

Treatment

Treatment is largely symptomatic and consists mainly of analgesic drugs and physical treatment. The application of heat to the neck is often very soothing and reduces muscle spasm. One of the most useful treatments is traction. This treatment aims to gently stretch the neck and again may be very soothing probably by decreasing muscle spasm. Traction may be performed manually or by a head harness with pulley and weights (Fig. 2.15). Weights used range from 6 to 10 lb. In severe cases admission to hospital for continuous traction may be indicated. Collars are a useful and inexpensive form of treatment. A soft collar made with felt and stockinette and worn as a muff at night probably works by keeping the tender area warm and can be very effective in relieving symptoms. When there is definite evidence of nerve root pressure, more substantial moulded collars made of plasterzote or polythene are indicated and these should be worn during the day as well as at night. Although it is usually possible by these means to alleviate symptoms, it is unlikely that they influence the course of the disease.

Manipulation can be used to alleviate cervical pain. It is most useful in the acute wry neck when it may produce early recovery.

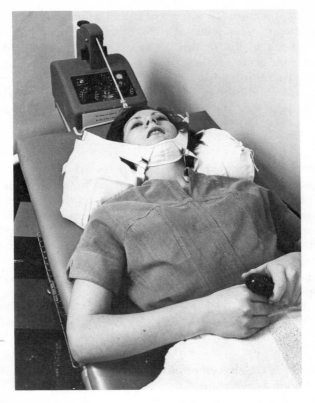

Fig. 2.15 Cervical traction using automated system.

Surgical removal of osteophytes impinging on nerve roots is very occasionally undertaken. In the syndrome of spinal stenosis caused by cord compression, surgery to relieve the pressure on the spinal cord is the only effective treatment.

Lumbar spondylosis and back pain

Osteoarthrosis of the lumbar spine is a common cause of back pain and the most well defined manifestation of spondylosis is the prolapsed intervertebral disc (PID). PID is a direct result of disc degeneration and prolapse does not occur in healthy discs. The lumbar and sacral nerve roots are particularly vulnerable to pressure from posterior and posterio-lateral bulging of prolapsed discs.

Prolapsed intervertebral disc (PID)

The onset of symptoms is usually sudden and typically follows a twisting movement or occurs if the patient overreaches himself in lifting. Although one might expect it to occur when lifting very heavy weights, movement and load may be trivial. Pain is usually felt immediately but is sometimes delayed. The patient may be unable to straighten up. If the damaged disc is pressing on a nerve root, pain will be experienced in the distribution of that root.

The lower lumbar and sacral roots are the most frequently affected and these cause pain radiating down the back of the thigh into the leg and foot. This pain is commonly called sciatica. Involvement of upper lumbar roots is less common and produces pain in the anterior thigh. Associated with this pain are the symptoms of nerve damage, ie paraesthesiae, numbness and weakness of affected musculature. The pain is worse on coughing, moving and sneezing. It is eased by lying supine and made worse by sitting and standing. Examination reveals considerable spasm of the paravertebral muscles with limitation and asymmetry of spinal movement. Neurological examination shows evidence of nerve damage depending on the nerve root involved. One of the most useful tests in PID is the straight leg raising test in which the patient lies flat on his back and the legs are passively lifted up in turn—this lifting produces stretching of the nerve plexus and the hamstring muscles. Normally people can straight leg raise to about 80–90°. If a nerve root is damaged by a disc, the straight leg raising test on that side will be correspondingly reduced, usually markedly so.

The natural course of events in acute PID is for the condition to gradually improve. Shrinking of the nucleus pulposus extrusion causes reduction of pressure on the nerve root and eventually full or partial neurological recovery occurs. Degenerate discs are inclined to repeat the performance and intermittent attacks may lead to more chronic forms of backache.

On the other hand, a central disc prolapse is a very serious condition indeed, as the prolapsed disc is extruded backwards into the cauda equina and many nerve roots may be involved, particularly the sacral roots, S2, 3 and 4. In this condition, as well as bilateral weakness of the legs, loss of sphincter control occurs with interference with micturition and defaecation.

Apophyseal osteoarthrosis

Apophyseal arthritis is commonly associated with disc disease. Most back pain probably comes from these joints and it may be difficult to distinguish a mild case of disc prolapse and nerve pressure from pain arising from these joints. Pain from these joints may radiate down the leg in a rather similar way to sciatica but is not made worse by manoeuvres which increase cerebro-spinal pressure, such as coughing and sneezing.

Spondylolisthesis and spondylisis

Spondylisis is a defect in the vertebral arch. When this defect is bilateral the vertebrae may slide forwards carrying the spinal column with them. This is then known as spondylolisthesis. Spondylolisthesis may also arise as a result of osteoarthrosis of the apophyseal joints. Patients usually present with chronic low back pain. If displacement is severe then the contents of the spinal canal, ie the nerve roots, are compressed and pain is felt down the leg and various degrees of nerve damage are evident.

Spinal stenosis

This is the term used to describe narrowing of the spinal canal causing pressure on the spinal cord or cauda equina. It is more likely to occur in people with a congenitally narrow canal. The ultimate cause of the narrowing may be a posterior lumbar disc protrusion or in the neck a posterior osteophyte growth. Narrowing may also occur due to distortion of bone such as occurs in Paget's disease or due to bony overgrowths associated with osteoarthrosis of the apophyseal joints. Achondroplasia is a congenital cause of spinal stenosis.

Clinically the nerve damage due to lumbar spinal stenosis results in a form of claudication with weakness and loss of sensation in the legs on walking, and relief on resting. If untreated, this can lead to loss of sphincter control and a flaccid paraplegia.

Structural back pain not due to spondylosis

There are other abnormalities which occur in the lumbar spine which may be a cause of back pain but are not necessarily associated with lumbar spondylosis.

Back pain, particularly dorsal pain in adolescents is sometimes due to Schuermann's disease. This is a developmental abnormality of the vertebral epiphysis which results in wedging of the dorsal vertebrae. In most people this abnormality is asymptomatic but a few present with intractable dorsal pain. Other causes of structural back pain are acute Schmorl's nodes occurring in young people after trauma; very small fractures impossible to see on conventional X-rays which should always be considered in acute back pain occurring in older people; congenital anomalies of the lower lumbar vertebrae also predispose to back pain.

Ankylosing hyperostosis is a condition characterized by gross osteophyte-like projections from the vertebrae which may fuse with projections from adjacent vertebrae, so completely stiffening segments of the spine. This is a harmless and usually incidental finding shown up only on X-ray.

Back pain without demonstrable structural cause

Patients are frequently seen in whom there is no radiological abnormality and diagnoses are made in terms of acute or chronic back strain. Because the methods of investigation are limited, the pathology in these cases is conjectural.

Bad posture is said to account for some chronic back pain and predisposes to acute attacks in others. This may be due to weak abdominal muscles due to repeated pregnancies and may result in hyper-lordosis and chronic low back pain. Unequal leg lengths produce scoliosis and possibly a tendency to back pain.

People who are more flexible than normal (hypermobile subjects) seem more prone to develop back pain which is probably secondary to ligamentous tears.

Back pain secondary to other diseases

Apart from the conditions listed above, the differential diagnosis of back pain also includes pain secondary to more serious diseases, see Table 2.1.

Investigations in back pain

The essential investigations are plain X-rays of the spine and simple blood tests such as an ESR. In osteoarthrosis and postural back pain, the ESR would be normal. In other conditions such as ankylosing

Table 2.1   Diseases Causing Back Pain

Bone disease	Osteoporosis *→ collapse v. us⁷ T vertex... suddler a sot pain*
	Osteomalacia
	Hyperparathyroidism
	Active Paget's disease of bone
Cancer	Myelomatosis
	Secondary tumours from breast, prostate, kidney, bronchus, etc.
Infections	T.B.
	Brucella
	Pyogenic infections
Ankylosing spondylitis	
Visceral causes	eg, pain arising from the kidney, pancreas and penetrating peptic ulcers

spondylitis, infection or cancer, it will usually be raised. Other blood tests and procedures are necessary to diagnose the conditions shown in the table.

If nerve root or cord pressure is suspected a myelogram (Fig. 2.16) or radiculogram is ordered. A lumbar puncture is carried out and a radio-opaque dye is inserted into the subarachnoid space. This dye outlines the structures within the spinal canal and it is possible to see areas of local pressure caused by a prolapsed intervertebral disc or a tumour. This investigation is essential to localize the site of neurological damage so that the surgeon knows which area to investigate. Myelography may be associated with considerable post lumbar puncture headache and sometimes an arachnoiditis occurs. To avoid this the radiologist removes the dye after the myelogram has been completed. Following a myelogram the patient should rest prone for at least twelve hours in order to avoid headache which is thought to be caused by cerebro-spinal fluid leaking from the lumbar puncture site.

The dye used in the radiculogram is more soluble than the dye used in a myelogram and it is not necessary to remove it from the spinal canal. However, it is very irritant to the brain and the patient has to remain in a seated position in bed after the procedure for 24 hours.

The treatment of lumbar spondylosis and back pain

Myth and magic abound in the treatment of back pain. This is due to the difficulty in obtaining an exact diagnosis in conditions other than

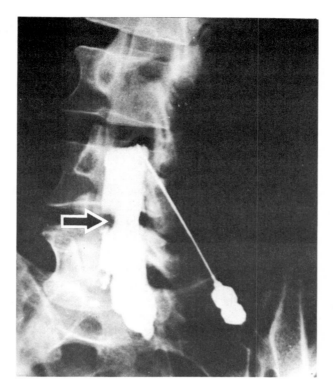

Fig. 2.16 A myelogram. The lumbar puncture needle is clearly seen. The spinal canal is outlined by the white contrast column, and indented by a prolapsed disc as shown by the black arrow.

that clearly relating to prolapsed intervertebral disc, and consequently because of the allied difficulty of testing treatments in the setting of a controlled clinical trial. Opinions are often held most strongly in the absence of facts.

Analgesics. Simple analgesics such as paracetamol one gram four hourly or Distalgesic one to two tablets four hourly, suffice for most causes of backache. However, an acute PID may be severely painful in the first few days and require stronger drugs such as Pentazocine or opiates like Pethidine.

Rest. Rest on a firm mattress is important for an acute PID. Pressure in lumbar discs is lowest in the supine position. The duration of rest will vary with the severity of symptoms and signs but four to six weeks should be adequate. If there has been no improvement after three weeks of rest, then surgery should be considered. Where bed rest is impossible, a plaster of Paris corset may provide adequate pain relief. Following bed rest it is advisable to wear a lumbo-sacral support, ie a corset, to restrict movement for a few months.

Corsets work by maintaining the lumbar lordosis and maintaining abdominal pressure, thus relieving the spine of excess weight. They also keep the back warm which helps in the winter but may be uncomfortable in a hot summer. Corsets restrict movement and if worn over long periods produce a stiff back which by itself is painful to move regardless of the initial pathology. Chronic back pain in the elderly and late middle aged where there is no hope of restoring posture or musculature may be much helped by surgical corsets and frequently here a corset is the only feasible treatment. Similarly, mild degrees of spondylolisthesis in this age group are also indications for the prescription of a corset. When dealing with old people it is important to ensure that they are able to put on and take off the corset themselves or that help is available for them to do this.

Traction. Lumbar traction by applying distracting forces on the lumbar vertebrae by means of a harness or weights is often helpful in relieving acute back pain and nerve root pain. It is doubtful whether it influences the course of the disease although an effect on bulging discs has been demonstrated radiologically. In the early stages of bed rest for acute PID lumbar traction is a very useful supplement.

Heat. Local heat is of value in temporarily relieving the muscle spasm associated with acute back pain. It has a similar temporary ameliorating effect on chronic back pain. The widespread use of liniments which are a method of applying local heat testify to the public satisfaction with this sort of treatment. Heat may be applied as infra-red heat, short-wave diathermy or by means of electrically heated pads.

Manipulation. Manipulation is a method of treatment where the operator attempts to alter the relative position of vertebrae by manual techniques. Various systems of such techniques have been described but those commonly used are the carefully graded movements described by Maitland and the rotatory methods described by Cyriax. Both these methods are usually carried out on the conscious patient but some orthopaedic surgeons admit people for manipulation under anaesthetic. Manipulation should not be applied in the presence of definite nerve root pressure but it may be of benefit in people with back pain without such complications. The clinical trial carried out by the British Association for Rheumatology and Rehabilitation showed no overall benefit from manipulation when comparing it with analgesics and the wearing of a corset. Nevertheless, the impression remains that a small group of patients with acute back pain do benefit from manipulation. The difficulty lies in identifying this small group of patients. It is important to realize that most cases of acute back pain will in any case get better spontaneously. The place of manipulation in the treatment of backache remains controversial but what is important is that the treatment is carried out by a properly qualified practitioner who is capable of distinguishing the possible causes of back pain and is aware of potential dangers in their treatment.

Exercises. Programmes of exercises are important both in the rehabilitation of acute PID and in the treatment of chronic postural back pain particularly in those with weak abdominal musculature and a hyper-lordosis. In this latter group the most useful exercises are abdominal flexion exercises designed to maintain and improve abdominal musculature. Exercises to mobilize stiff spines, particularly after acute PID and operations for PID or following corset incarceration, may be made more effective if carried out in a hydrotherapy pool.

Other non-surgical methods. In some Centres acute back pain is treated by epidural injections of hydrocortisone and a local anaesthetic. In others, prolapsed intervertebral discs have been treated by injection of an enzyme (Papain) into the nucleus pulposus which destroys the disc.

Surgery. The chief place of surgery in osteoarthrosis of the spine is in relieving pressure on the spinal cord and nerves. Operations vary from excising the prolapsed part of the nucleus pulposus to removing sections of the vertebral arch to relieve pressure on the cord or cauda equina. Sometimes a surgeon may remove osteophytes which are pressing on a cervical nerve root. An unstable spinal segment such as occurs in spondylolisthesis may require fusion of the unstable part to adjoining vertebrae.

Rehabilitation of patients with backache

The general principles of rehabilitation are covered in Chapter 17. Back injuries and spinal osteoarthrosis are common amongst workers in heavy industry and these men often present a particularly difficult problem in rehabilitation as their back pain precludes them from their previous employment. They may be poorly educated with a limited ability to adapt to different forms of employment. The role of the Disablement Resettlement Officer and the Employment Rehabilitation Centres are very important here.

Recovery from back pain can be greatly influenced by psychological illness and it is very important when treating patients with back pain that specific enquiry be made for symptoms of psychological disease such as sleep disturbances, anorexia and loss of libido. Recovery will be delayed until the psychological problem is investigated and treated.

Further reading

Jayson, M. I. V. (ed.). *The Lumbar Spine and Back Pain*. Sector Publishing Ltd.

Wright, Verna (ed.). *Osteoarthrosis*. In series *Clinics in Rheumatic Diseases*. W. B. Saunders & Co. Ltd.

3
Rheumatoid Arthritis

Rheumatoid arthritis (RA) is the commonest type of inflammatory arthritis. It is a disease which may affect other parts of the body apart from the joints and for this reason it is sometimes known as rheumatoid disease.

There is no precise definition of the disease, diagnosis depending on the presence of certain criteria, described below.

Criteria for Rheumatoid Arthritis

1. A peripheral symmetrical arthritis
2. Nodules
3. Bony erosions on X-ray
4. Rheumatoid factor in the blood

---

1. RA is often described as a peripheral symmetrical arthritis, peripheral because the small joints of the hands and feet are involved and symmetrical because both sides of the body are affected. Any synovial tissue can be involved. However, it must be pointed out that in about 20% of cases the onset of the disease is not symmetrical.

2. Nodules may be present. These can be found in the skin, attached to bones or tendons, or in other parts of the body, particularly those areas subject to pressure, eg the elbows. The nodules have a characteristic structure when examined histologically.

3. The disease causes destruction of bone at the edge of the joints; this loss of bone is visible on X-ray and is called an erosion (Fig. 3.1).

4. Blood from patients with rheumatoid arthritis may contain an antibody called rheumatoid factor. This is found using the Latex or sheep cell agglutination test (SCAT). If the test is positive the disease is then referred to as sero-positive rheumatoid arthritis, and if negative, sero-negative rheumatoid arthritis. This test for rheumatoid factor is important in diagnosis and in determining the prognosis. Rheumatoid factor, however, may also occur in normal people especially in the elderly and in diseases other than rheumatoid arthritis.

If all these criteria are met, the patient has rheumatoid arthritis.

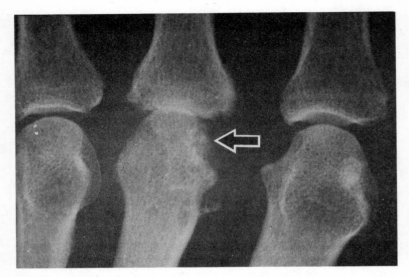

Fig. 3.1 Middle joint shows rheumatoid erosion (arrow). Note also that the joint space is lost in this joint.

However, many people do not have all these criteria and then diagnosis may be more difficult.

Epidemiology

Because there is no definite test for rheumatoid arthritis, it is not easy to decide how many people in a community have the disease. However, there is no doubt that women seem to be affected two or three times as often as men. On average, about one person in every hundred has definite rheumatoid arthritis. Similar figures are present for all parts of the world. Climate, dampness and social status do not seem to have any bearing on the chances of having the disease.

Table 3.1 Percentage of Population with Definite Rheumatoid Arthritis

Area of survey	Males	Females	Both
Wensleydale–Leigh (England)	0.47	1.6	1.07
Rotterdam (Holland)	0.5	1.2	
Michigan (U.S.A.)	0.3	0.7	0.5
Puerto Rico	0.16	0.4	0.34
Japan	0.4	0.7	0.55

Aetiology

Although the cause of the disease is unknown, many ideas have been put forward and explored. These may be grouped under the following headings:

1. Heredity. Hereditary factors do seem to have a modest influence on the chance of contracting rheumatoid arthritis. Some studies suggest that relatives of rheumatoid patients have an increased chance of developing the disease and recently genetic differences have been shown between groups of people with and without rheumatoid arthritis.

2. Infection. Several viral infections, eg german measles (rubella), and serum hepatitis may produce a transient arthritis similar to rheumatoid disease and it is possible that RA may begin as such a viral infection. There are analogies in veterinary medicine where an infective arthritis of pigs shows similarities to RA. Thorough searches have been made for an infective agent and several types of organisms have from time to time been isolated from rheumatoid joints, eg mycoplasma. However, these experiments have not produced consistent results and there is still no firm evidence that any of these organisms is instrumental in causing the disease and certainly no single causative microbe has been isolated so far.

3. Altered immunity. In rheumatoid joints there is evidence of an active immunological process. The lining of the joint is infiltrated by lymphocytes and plasma cells. Both types of cells are essential in fighting infection, but in the rheumatoid joint their activities appear to be deleterious to the joint itself. This is most clearly seen with plasma cells which produce rheumatoid factor, an antibody which combines with the patient's own globulin. This combination occurring within the joint results in an inflammation which is instrumental in causing joint destruction.

This state of affairs can be initiated in rabbits by injecting minute amounts of foreign protein into their joints. It is conceivable, therefore, that a circulating foreign protein, perhaps a virus located in a person's joints, sets up an active immunological process which whilst being directed initially against the organism results in joint destruction as a side effect.

4. Psychosocial factors. There is no evidence to suggest that any particular personality type is prone to rheumatoid arthritis. It does seem possible that in some cases psychological stress may precipitate the disease.

5. Trauma. Controlled surveys have never demonstrated that trauma to a joint is the cause of rheumatoid arthritis. Nevertheless occasionally patients are seen in whom the event intitiating the disease appears to be injury to a particular joint.

Pathology

Although rheumatoid arthritis can affect many systems in the body, the brunt of the disease, certainly in the majority of cases, falls on the joints, and in this section we will deal exclusively with the effect of the disease on the joints.

1. Swelling of the joint occurs first mainly because of swelling and

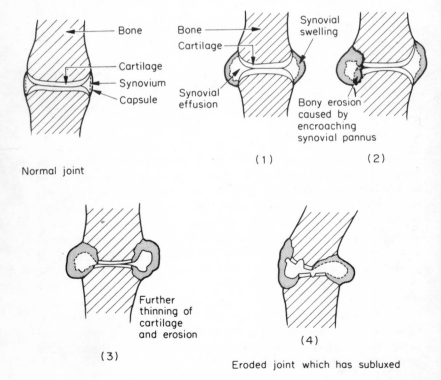

Fig. 3.2 Pathology of rheumatoid arthritis stages (1) to (4). Diagrammatic section through joints.

increasing size of the synovium. The synovium exudes more fluid than normal and produces an effusion contributing to the joint swelling. This effusion contains numerous white cells which are lymphocytes at first and later polymorphonucleocytes. The effusion has a high protein content. See Fig. 3.2(1).

2. Progressive swelling and growth of the synovium begins to encroach upon the cartilage at the edge of the joint. This encroaching synovium is called a pannus. The encroaching pannus results in the destruction of bone and cartilage and produces the characteristic X-ray erosion. See Fig. 3.2(2).

3. At the same time, enzymes released from white blood cells breaking down within the synovial cavity damage other parts of the joint cartilage. The result may be total destruction of the joint surfaces with weakening of ligaments and joint capsule. See Fig. 3.2(3).

4. This leads to instability of the joint, subluxation and even complete dislocation. Further progress may produce fibrous or bony fusion with stiffness or complete rigidity of the joint. See Fig. 3.2(4).

The progress of the disease may halt at any of these stages.

If the joint mobility is maintained, the damage to the joint may result in secondary osteoarthritis.

Clinical features of rheumatoid arthritis (general)

The onset of the disease is usually insiduous with the appearance of pain, swelling and morning stiffness particularly of the small peripheral joints. Numbness and tingling in the hands may be associated with increasing tightness of wedding rings, which have to be removed. Pain may often be felt first in the forefeet. In about 20% of cases, the onset of the disease is more sudden with pronounced joint pain, swelling and general malaise; a fever may be present.

The disease may start as a monarthritis particularly of the knee and in fact at least 30% of patients with rheumatoid arthritis do begin with involvement of the proximal joints.

The disease may sometimes be preceded by a period of general ill health characterized by anorexia, weight loss, easy fatigue and paraesthesia. In other patients rheumatoid arthritis may be preceded by the condition known as palindromic rheumatism (see Chapter 12, p. 152).

There is a tendency for the disease to start in the winter months.

The course of rheumatoid arthritis may be divided broadly into two phases, the early and the late. In the early phase of disease, symptoms are due mainly to active inflammation of the joints, whereas in the late phase the symptoms are due to secondary osteo-arthritis and deformity.

Pain is the most serious and constant symptom. It comes initially from the effects of inflammation and swelling in much the same way as a boil is painful. It may keep the patient awake at night, and be worse in the morning on getting up. Exercising the affected joint excessively makes the pain worse, although gentle exercise is often beneficial in overcoming stiffness. Later in the course of the disease, joint pain may arise from secondary osteoarthritis and in this con-dition it is almost entirely related to exercise and may not be associ-ated with morning exacerbations and stiffness.

In the active inflammatory phase stiffness is felt in joints and muscles particularly in the morning and after sitting or resting for a time. Morning stiffness is an indicator of disease activity and may last from hours to all day. This is a serious disability for people engaged in active work in the home or outside. It may mean getting up hours before normal so that the daily chores of dressing and washing can be completed on time.

Local joint stiffness of a more permanent type may be the result of scarring of the joint capsule (a contracture) occurring after many bouts of inflammation.

Early onset of fatigue is another feature of rheumatoid arthritis unrelated to pain. For this reason it is often a good idea to advise an afternoon rest period. One must also take this tendency to tire easily into account when considering a person's ability to return to full-time work.

Symptoms may also arise from the systemic features of rheumatoid arthritis such as involvement of the eye, nerves, blood vessels and lungs.

Clinical features of articular manifestations

1. Hands. Deviation of the fingers towards the ulnar (little finger) side of the hand commonly occurs in RA (Fig. 3.3) with subluxation of the metacarpo-phalangeal joints and slipping of the extensor tendons off the top of the joints to the ulnar side. Ulnar deviation does not cause a great loss of function but may be unsightly.

Swan necking of fingers on the other hand, produces a hand unable to grasp. There is extreme and eventually fixed extension at the proximal interphalangeal joint and a compensatory flexion at the

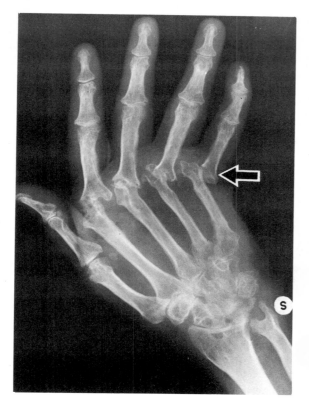

Fig. 3.3 Ulnar deviation in advanced RA. Arrow points to dislocated, eroded MCP joint. Note the erosion of the lower end of ulna(S).

terminal interphalangeal joint. In the early stages this is reversible by splintage but later improvement can only be achieved surgically.

Buttonhole (Boutonnière) deformities (Fig. 3.4) are the opposite of swan necking and are produced by hyperflexion of the PIP joint and extension of the TIPs. They are so called because the extensor tendon splits around the joint which pokes through it, the split tendon resembling a buttonhole.

Loss of hand function is also caused by inflammation, fibrosis and tightening of the capsules of the small joints of the hands producing stiffness. The synovial covering of the flexor tendons in the hands may become inflamed and thickened and obstruct the easy sliding of tendons up and down the fibrous canal on the volar surface of the fingers. This prevents full finger flexion. The thickening

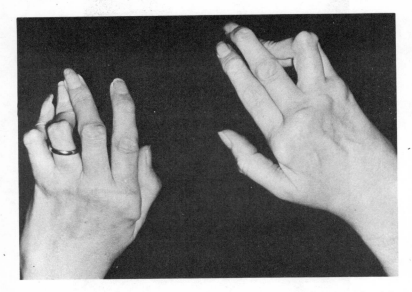

Fig. 3.4   The outer three fingers on the left hand and outer two on the right show Boutonnière deformities.

of the synovial lining may be palpable in the hands as nodular thickenings.

2. Wrists. The wrist is very commonly affected in rheumatoid arthritis. Very early on in the disease the lower end of the ulna becomes more prominent and erosion of this bone (Fig. 3.3) produces both local pain and tenderness and may cause rupture of extensor tendons passing over it. Restriction of the wrist is common and sometimes associated with subluxation.

3. Elbows. Involvement of the elbows soon produces flexion deformities with inability to extend the elbow fully. Radio-ulnar arthritis at the elbow results in pain on pronation and supination and eventually loss of movement as well.

4. Shoulders. Pain and restriction of movement at the shoulder joint is common and due to inflammation and subsequent scarring of the gleno-humeral joint. Movement of the shoulder then takes place mainly at the thoracic scapular level. Arthritis of the acromio-clavicular joint will also cause pain and restriction of shoulder movement.

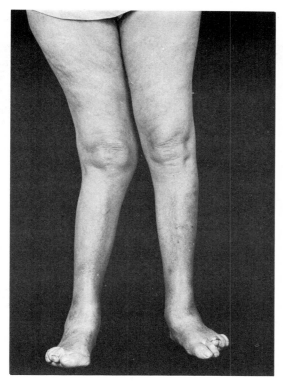

Fig. 3.5 RA of the knee causing instability and marked genu valgum of the right knee.

5. Hips. The hip joint may become eroded and destroyed like any other synovial joint. Pain due to hip involvement is felt principally in the groin, thigh, buttock and knee. Flexion deformities are common. Sometimes the femoral head may die and disintegrate; this is known as aseptic necrosis. The femoral head may also progress towards the pelvis with the acetabulum being pushed before it. This is called protrusio acetabulare and is a particular feature of inflammatory arthritis of the hip joint (see Fig. 16.4).

6. Knees. The particular feature of knee involvement is the occurrence of instability due to laxity and destruction of ligaments or due to loss of bone (Fig. 3.5).

Another frequent feature of an active synovitis of the knee is the appearance of popliteal cysts due to the production of large amounts of fluid within the knee causing backward pressure on the joint capsule (Fig. 3.6). These cysts may become very large and extend down into the calf. On occasions they may rupture and produce

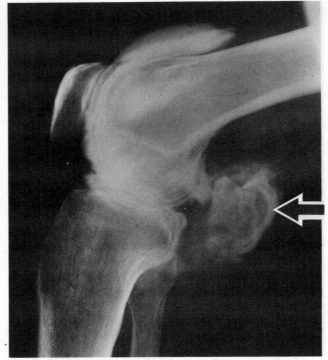

Fig. 3.6 Arthrogram of the knee joint. A popliteal cyst (arrowed) has formed behind the knee joint.

sudden pain and swelling of the calf. This may be confused with a deep vein thrombosis but the treatment is entirely different.

7. Feet. The most common disorder of the feet is inflammation and subluxation of the metatarso–phalangeal joints (MTP). The subluxation is upwards producing clawing of the toes (Fig. 3.7).

The skin under the subluxed joints becomes thickened to form calluses (Fig. 3.8). This sensation is likened to walking on marbles.

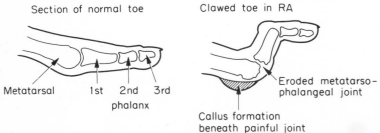

Fig. 3.7 Clawing of the toes in RA (see also top of facing page 45).

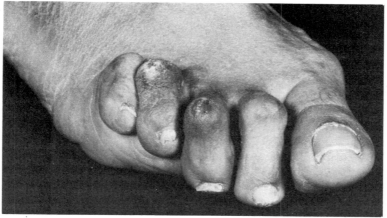

Fig. 3.7 *(Continued)*
The arthritis may also affect the ankle joint producing pain and reduced movement at this joint especially on walking. Involvement of the sub-talar and tarsal joints commonly produces a stiff flat foot with a valgus heel deformity.

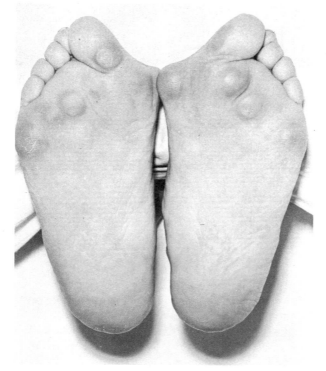

Fig. 3.8 Callosities on the forefeet in rheumatoid arthritis.

8. Neck. Although rheumatoid arthritis is principally an arthritis of peripheral joints, the neck is often involved. This involvement is important because dislocation of vertebrae in the neck due to rheumatoid arthritis may cause compression of the cervical cord and even death. About 30% of hospital in-patients have some degree of cervical instability due to their rheumatoid arthritis. The odontoid

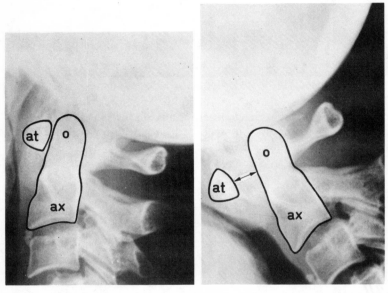

Fig. 3.9   The X-ray on the left is taken in extension and shows the normal position of the odontoid peg (o) closely applied to the anterior arch of the atlas (αt). (ax) axis. The film in (b) on the right is of the same patient taken with the neck flexed. There is abnormal movement (arrow) between the atlas and odontoid peg, endangering the spinal cord which lies immediately behind the odontoid peg.

peg of the second cervical vertebra, the axis, is normally held in place by the transverse ligament which passes behind it. Inflammation of the small synovial layer between the ligament and the odontoid peg may weaken the ligament and allow undue movement of the odontoid peg. This is most evident in forward flexion of the neck (Fig. 3.9) and if the movement is very excessive, compression of the spinal cord may take place as it leaves the skull. Compression of the spinal cord may also take place lower down as small joints in the lower cervical spine known as the neurocentral joints may also become affected by arthritis and produce so much inflammation and destruction that the lower cervical vertebrae may slip out of place resulting in damage to the cervical cord. In both instances subluxation or dislocation of cervical vertebrae should be readily visible on X-ray especially if films are taken with the patient's head in flexion.

It is important before any rheumatoid patient goes to theatre for an operation that an X-ray of the neck be taken to rule out possible subluxation of the cervical vertebrae.

9. Tendons. Tendons frequently become involved in rheumatoid arthritis. Rheumatoid nodules form on the Achilles tendon behind the heel and over the fingers and tendons split resulting in Boutonnière finger deformities.

Inflammation of the flexor tendon sheaths in the hand cause nodular swellings which result in the syndrome of trigger finger.

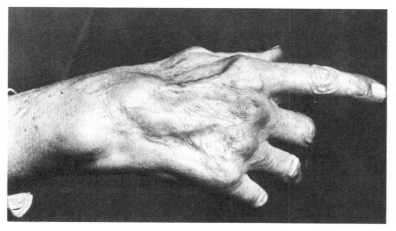

Fig. 3.10 The outer three fingers are drooping because the extensor tendons on the back of the hand have ruptured.

The most dramatic tendon disease is attrition rupture which occurs to the extensor tendons of the fingers as they pass over a roughened lower end of ulna. This results in the sudden inability to lift the affected fingers (Fig. 3.10). Surgical repair is the only effective treatment.

Diagnosis

Diagnosis is essentially made on the strength of the history and clinical examination. Blood should be taken for a full blood count,

ESR, and examination made for SCAT and Latex tests. In rheumatoid arthritis the ESR will almost invariably be raised and mild anaemia will often be present. The white cell count and platelet count are usually within normal limits unless complications are present such as an arteritis or Felty's syndrome (see systemic manifestations, p. 58). In typical cases the Latex and SCAT tests will be positive. Liver function tests may demonstrate a raised alkaline phosphatase which is frequently found in rheumatoid arthritis, a serum bilirubin and transaminases are normal. A serum iron and IBC will normally both be low, a feature of any generalized inflammatory illness. In a typical case X-rays of the hands and feet will show erosions and it is important always to X-ray the feet in suspected cases of rheumatoid arthritis as asymptomatic MTP erosions are sometimes found. In cases presenting as a monarthritis, synovial biopsy may be necessary to distinguish this from an infection such as tuberculosis.

Course and Prognosis

The usual course of events is for the disease to come and go over a number of years with slow and gradual progression. Complete remissions may sometimes last for many years and it is because the course of the disease is so unpredictable that it is so difficult to assess the value of treatments. There are a few patients who after an initial often acute onset have no more trouble. On the other hand, other patients may progress rapidly to complete crippling in less than five years from starting the disease. It must be emphasized that in hospital one sees the worst disease and that in the community there are cases of milder disease which never come to hospital or even to the general practitioner.

Surveys of hospital patients carried out show that of a typical group at the end of ten years from original admission approximately 20% would be completely independent in all ways, whereas about 10% would be completely crippled and dependent. The remainder fall between these two extremes. Factors identified as influencing prognosis adversely are early symmetrical involvement of joints, a long interval between the onset of the disease and admission to hospital, an insidious onset rather than acute onset and a positive SCAT test. In general, women appear to do rather worse than men initially and older people worse than younger.

Factors adversely affecting prognosis

1. Insidious onset
2. Age
3. Early symmetrical arthritis
4. Late presentation at clinic
5. Positive SCAT test
6. Female sex

Patients with rheumatoid arthritis die from the same diseases as the normal population but have a slightly higher death rate.

Management of Rheumatoid Arthritis

There being no cure for rheumatoid arthritis, the objects of treatment are to suppress the disease where possible, this is often called inducing a remission; to reduce inflammation and pain; to reduce joint destruction and avoid deformities and to overcome physical and social handicaps.

Objects of Treatment

1. Reduce pain
2. Reduce joint destruction
3. Avoid deformities
4. Overcome, and adjust to, disability and handicap

The chief means of treatment are rest, drugs and splintage. To these we might also add controlled exercise, occupational therapy and counselling.

Rest. Rest may be applied locally or generally. Rest subserves the first three of our objects of treatment. Pain is relieved by rest and probably joint destruction is lessened by the lack of trauma thereby reducing the likelihood of deformities.

General bed rest means no weight bearing. Emphasis on the good position in bed is essential (see Chapter 15, p. 181). It is best for morale if the patients can use the normal lavatory but they should be conveyed there in wheelchairs. The duration of bed rest is controversial but in general patients should be rested until lower limb joint pains are absent on attempted weight bearing. This is a counsel of perfection and has to be weighed against the complications of bed rest. The complications of prolonged bed rest are loss of bone from the skeleton (disuse osteoporosis), the tendency to develop renal calculi, wasting of muscle and consequent loss of muscle power. These complications can be at least partially obviated by in-bed exercises.

However, the social complications of prolonged in-patient care such as the effect on the marriage and the family unit, are more difficult to deal with and are perhaps the most telling complications of prolonged hospital care. One must also bear in mind the expense of in-patient care.

Nevertheless, patients with active arthritis do benefit from a period of bed rest and bearing the above strictures in mind should be offered it.

Drugs. Drugs used in rheumatoid arthritis may be divided into two groups, first and second line drugs.

First Line Drugs
Analgesics: Paracetamol
                                         Dextropropoxyphene
                                         Codeine
Anti-inflammatory analgesics: Aspirin, 3.6–4.8 g*
                                         Ibuprofen, 1200 mg*
                                         Indomethacin, 150–200 mg*
                                         Naproxen, 500–1000 mg*
                                         Ketoprofen, 100–200 mg*
                                         Fenoprofen, 900–2400 mg*
                                         and others

Local intra-articular corticosteroid injections;
eg hydrocortisone acetate, methylprednisolone acetate,
triamcinolone

Second Line Drugs
Systemic corticosteroids, eg prednisolone or ACTH
Chloroquine
Gold
Penicillamine
Levamisole
Azathioprine
Cyclophosphamide

* *Dose in RA in 24 hours*

First line drugs are used to stop pain. The anti-inflammatory analgesics are more effective than the pure analgesics because inflammation itself is a potent cause of pain in rheumatoid arthritis. However,
as far as we know they do not reduce joint destruction although their
use does enable a rheumatoid patient to carry on with a normal life
and life would be unthinkable without such drugs for most
rheumatoid patients.

Aspirin is the most commonly used analgesic of this class and best
given as enteric coated tablets to avoid dyspepsia, in a dose of 3.6 to
4.8 g per day.

Indomethacin is often given by mouth or as a 100 mg, rectal
suppository at night to overcome morning stiffness. An alternative
here is naproxen 500 mg, by mouth or suppository at night before
retiring.

As seen in the list above (see also Chapter 14) there are many
alternatives each with their own advantages and disadvantages. In
practice, it has been found that there is much individual variation in
response to these drugs and individuals often do better on one
particular drug rather than another. The choice must be made by trial
and error.

Second line drugs are used when simple treatment such as rest and
first line drugs fail. Apart from corticosteroids these drugs have a
delayed effect, ie the patient will notice no difference in his state for
up to three months after the start of treatment. After this delay there
is a variable and progressive improvement in joint pain, swelling and
general health and a fall in the ESR. This improvement is known as a
remission. However, all these drugs entail the possibility of severe
side effects and for this reason are given only to moderately and
severely affected people and careful monitoring is needed, preferably
in special clinics.

The remission usually lasts for a variable time after stopping the
drug. It is not clear whether these drugs affect the course of the
disease but there is evidence that gold reduces joint destruction and
penicillamine possibly prevents the progression of palindromic
rheumatism to rheumatoid arthritis.

In contrast to other second line drugs, corticosteroids act immediately to reduce inflammation, stiffness and pain. They are usually
given as prednisolone or enteric coated prednisolone in doses of up to
10 mg per day in joint problems, but in higher doses for some of the
systemic features of rheumatoid arthritis such as vasculitis and
neuropathy. Their effect is often dramatic but because of their
efficacy it is often extremely difficult to wean people off them. This

should be attempted because of the far-reaching side effects of these drugs. The indications for steroid treatment are:

    (1) Failure to respond to adequate conservative treatment plus a second line drug such as gold.

    (2) Systemic disease.

    (3) Economic and or social reasons, eg a small dose of prednisolone sometimes tides patients over a difficult time at work and avoids unemployment through frequent sick leave absence.

They can also be given in the intervals between starting a second line drug and the onset of the remission and then tailed off when the remission occurs. In addition steroids are effective in treating many of the side effects of second line drugs such as thrombocytopaenia and dermatitis.

Local steroid injections particularly into inflamed joints have a very important place. They are used to supplement the conservative regimen, first line drugs and splintage. They are given as hydrocortisone acetate or methylprednisolone acetate. They usually produce a dramatic reduction in the signs of inflammation and the beneficial effect lasts from days to weeks. Possible complications of local steroid injections are:

    (1) Infection introduced by the injection.

    (2) Damaged cartilage especially if the injections are too frequent and the dose is too high.

    (3) Post-injection flare of the arthritis.

    (4) Systemic steroid effect if the injections are too frequent.

In fact, infection although a possibility is rare in practice. In one series only 1 in 14 000 injections resulted in joint infection. Damage to cartilage is more a theoretical than a practical complication but it is wise to avoid trauma to the joint, such as weight bearing, for 24 hours after the injection. A post-injection flare is not uncommon and usually lasts for a few hours and then subsides.

The precautions necessary for the use of intra-articular steroids are as follows:

    (1) Ensure first that there is no infection in the joint. This may require aspiration and culture of synovial fluid before injection can take place.

    (2) Use a sterile non-touch technique.

    (3) Multidose vials should not be used more than once.

The joints most often injected are not surprisingly those that can most easily be entered with a needle. These are the knees, shoulders, wrists, elbows and metacarpo-phalangeal joints. Rheumatoid tendonitis can also be treated with local steroid injections.

Radio-active synovectomy. Over the last few years it has become the practice in many Centres to instil radio-active isotopes into joints in an attempt to destroy the rheumatoid synovium. The most common joint treated in this way is the knee and the most common isotope used is Yttrium 90. The procedure is performed with full precautions under the direction of a radiotherapist. At the moment this treatment would seem to be an effective alternative in many cases to surgical synovectomy. Because the long-term effect of instillation of radio-active isotopes into joints is unknown, this procedure is limited to older patients at present.

The treatment of local joint disease

Hands. Rest splints usually made of plaster of Paris are used in the acute stage to rest painful wrists and hands in a good position in hospital. Splints like these can continue to be used at home especially at night. Local steroid injections into the wrists and MCP joints are useful at this stage. Later, polythene work splints can be made to support the wrist in action. These splints tend to be rather bulky and the provision of a soft palmar section improves the patient's grip and feel whilst wearing them. The ability to form a fist and grip can be improved by local steroid injection of the flexor tendon sheaths, by the wearing of a corrective splint and by local hand exercises such as squeezing of a latex ball.

Where flexion contractures are present passive stretching exercises may be usefully combined with the application of sequential plaster of Paris palmar shells. There are a number of surgical operations that may be used on the hand and the wrist, the most useful of which is removal of an eroded lower end of the ulna with synovectomy of the wrist. Synovectomy and joint replacement of the small joints of the hands have a limited place and are described in Chapter 16. In these latter operations intensive and well-planned post-operative physiotherapy is essential.

Elbow. The elbow can be splinted but this is commonly not done. The most useful local measure to correct flexion contractures at the elbow is local steroid injections, which are effective if there is active synovitis present. Surgical removal of the radial head and synovectomy improves the range of movement and decreases pain.

Shoulder. Restriction of shoulder movement and pain arises both from the acromio-clavicular joint and disease of the gleno-humeral joint. Local steroid injections into these joints are a useful preliminary to active exercises with or without slings to increase the range of movement.

Neck. The problems of pain arising from rheumatoid arthritis in the neck are handled mainly by immobilization. Collars range from soft collars to moulded plastic or block leather types (Fig. 3.11). None of

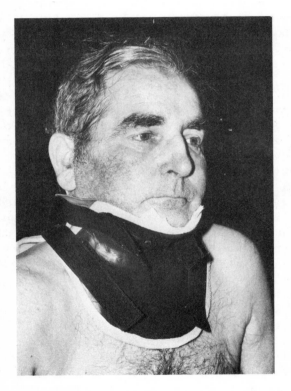

Fig. 3.11 Block leather collar in patient with rheumatoid neck.

these collars provide complete immobilization and the more rigid ones are cumbersome to wear. Continuous light traction with a head harness in hospital can provide relief of pain. If there is cervical subluxation and neurological complications such as nerve root or spinal cord damage, then it is necessary to immobilize the neck and reduce subluxation by use of skull traction with Crutchfield tongs preferably on a Striker frame. A more permanent fixation of the subluxed cervical segments can then be obtained by surgical fusion.

Hips. Hip pain can be relieved, at least temporarily, by bed rest and if necessary supplemented by skin traction. Fixed flexion contractures can be improved by periods of prone lying, non-weight-bearing exercises in the hydrotherapy pool, or the use of slings can improve the range of painfree movement. Local steroid injections are very difficult to locate accurately and so have little place. Benefit from these procedures is usually only temporary. Fortunately the success of total hip replacement has provided a solution to those rheumatoid patients with moderate to severe pain and disability from hip involvement.

Knees. When there is active synovitis present, a period of rest in a gutter splint is useful. The knee can also be immobilized in a plaster of Paris cylinder which can later be split longitudinally (bivalved) and used as a rest splint. The knee joint is easy to enter with a needle and synovitis of this joint can simply be ameliorated by aspiration and local steroid injections with or without a period of rest and splinting. Wasting of the quadriceps muscles is a feature of arthritis of the knee and exercises to strengthen these muscles are an important part in any treatment programme. These exercises improve the stability of the joint. The exercises may be static in which case they can be performed in bed even when the knee is in a plaster cylinder, or performed against resistance using manual pressure or weights. Kicking quadriceps exercises performed whilst sitting on the side of the bed also serve to reduce fixed flexion contractures. Flexion contractures of the knee can also be tackled by serial splinting whereby progressively straighter plaster cylinders are applied.

Instability of the knee can be ameliorated by the use of removable plastic cylinders or in some cases by the use of full length calipers. Before prescribing this type of appliance, however, one must be certain that the patient can cope with the appliance at home.

Synovectomy of the knee is a procedure which has been shown to reduce the progression of the disease in the operated joint. It is best to perform it when there is only minor damage. Other operations which are done for arthritis of the knee are tibial osteotomy which relieves pain, and various methods of joint replacement which aim to provide new bearing surfaces for the knee joint.

The treatment of a popliteal cyst is first to rest the knee, aspirate it and inject with local steroid. If the cyst does not decrease or recurs, then anterior synovectomy is the treatment of choice. 'Synovectomy' of the knee can be performed using a radio-active isotope which is injected into the knee. This is an alternative to surgical removal of the synovium.

The foot. The problem of MTP subluxation and callus formation can be dealt with in a number of ways. Simple paring of the callosity can reduce discomfort but this has to be repeated. The wearing of pads which lie just behind the MTP heads takes some of the weight off the MTP joint (Fig. 3.12). An alternative is the application of a

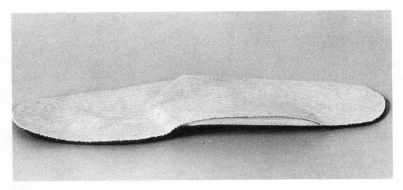

Fig. 3.12   Supportive insole.

transverse metatarsal bar to the shoe of the patient. Finally the other non-surgical approach is to provide surgical shoes; there are different ways of making these shoes but the principle is that the shoe is modelled to the sole of the foot so that body weight is well distributed over the sole of the foot and every part of the foot is well supported.

In many patients, Fowler's operation, where the painful metatarso-phalangeal joints are excised, produces an excellent result and obviates the need for modified footwear.

A painful ankle can be treated by a period of non-weight bearing and local steroid injections. A painful ankle can also be helped by wearing supportive ankle boots rather than shoes. The development of a stiff flat foot and a valgus heel deformity commonly produces symptoms in patients with rheumatoid arthritis. The discomfort can be helped by the wearing of a long arch support or by further modifications to the shoes. A below-knee caliper will stabilize a painful ankle and hind foot and is found useful by many patients despite the cosmetic problems. Operations to stiffen the hind foot (triple arthrodesis) are possible, but rarely used. Recently an artificial ankle joint has been developed but its place in treatment is still undetermined.

Occupational Therapy

This is an important feature in the treatment of rheumatoid arthritis and ideally all patients with rheumatoid arthritis should at least be interviewed by an occupational therapist. The chief purpose of occupational therapy now is to assess the patient's performance of everyday tasks and to analyse the nature and extent of the handicap. The occupational therapist is then in a position to advise on alternative methods of performance and to recommend aids and if necessary adaptations to the home. The assessment ideally takes place both in an Occupational Therapy Unit and with follow-up in a patient's home.

In many units the occupational therapist is responsible for the manufacture of more complicated types of splints used in rheumatoid arthritis.

Social Work and Counselling.

A chronic painful disabling condition like rheumatoid arthritis has tremendous impact on the victim's ability to cope with everyday problems of living, both domestic and at work. There is a profound effect on personal and family relationships. Conversely, depression arising from failure to resolve these problems will adversely affect the response of the patient to treatment. For these reasons a social worker is an important member of the therapeutic team as her interviews with the patient should bring these problems to light. In addition the medical social worker's expertise is important in making sure that the patient obtains available welfare benefits.

Nurses, because of their close contact with patients in hospital, are often in an ideal position to discover domestic and social difficulties which are worrying their patients. Patients should then be encouraged to disclose their problems to the consultant or social worker.

The ward sister will frequently see the patient's relatives and will be in a position to resolve personal problems herself particularly if they arise from ignorance about the disease, as is often the case. Her observations on the relationships between the patient and family are valuable in the total assessment of the patient.

Finally, the ARC handbooks on arthritis, and arthritis, sex and marriage, should be made available to all patients with rheumatoid arthritis.

The Systemic Features of Rheumatoid Arthritis

One of the important facts about rheumatoid arthritis is that the disease affects other parts of the body besides the joints. Many of these so-called systemic features of the disease are uncommon but a few such as anaemia are very common. Occasionally patients present primarily with a systemic complication rather than arthritis, eg they may present with rheumatoid inflammation of the eye.

Systemic features	
Nodules	Lung nodules
Anaemia	Sjogren's syndrome
Pericarditis	Scleritis
Arteritis	Keratomalacia
Neuropathy	Felty's syndrome
Pleural effusion	2^e Amyloidosis
Pulmonary fibrosis	Liability to infections

Nodules

These occur in about 20% of patients with rheumatoid arthritis. They occur mainly over pressure areas such as elbows (Fig. 3.13), and are definitely related to trauma. There is a characteristic histology. Nodules may cavitate, discharge or become infected. They can, if necessary, be removed surgically.

Anaemia

Anaemia is very common in active rheumatoid arthritis. In one series more than one out of five women with active disease had haemoglobins of less than 70%. This anaemia may be due to a number of causes. In active rheumatoid arthritis there is an inability of the bone marrow to produce enough red cells and although iron is absorbed normally by rheumatoid patients they are not able to utilize it

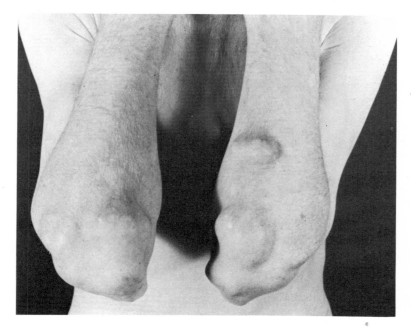

Fig. 3.13 Rheumatoid nodules in characteristic site.

properly for the production of haemoglobin and it tends to remain in iron stores instead of finding its way into the red cells. Cortisone dramatically reverses this disorder and causes an increase in haemoglobin. There is also a slightly increased breakdown of red cells in rheumatoid arthritis. The anaemia of rheumatoid arthritis responds to treatment of the disease, eg gold.

In some patients chronic blood loss from aspirin and similar drugs which cause bleeding from the gut may be an important factor.

Arteritis

Rheumatoid disease is one of the causes of arterial inflammation or arteritis. Inflammation of small arteries results in blocking of the arterial lumen. This in turn results in death of the area of tissue that the artery supplies. This dead tissue is known as an infarct. In RA these infarcts are most easily visible as black specks alongside finger nails (nail fold lesions, Fig. 3.14). This sort of arteritis is often associated with leg ulcers. Occasionally whole digits can become gangrenous (Fig. 3.15).

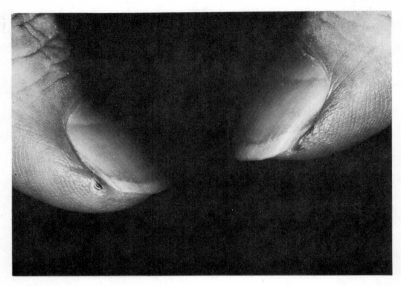

Fig. 3.14   Nail-fold lesions.

Fig. 3.15   More extensive infection causing gangrene of tip of finger.

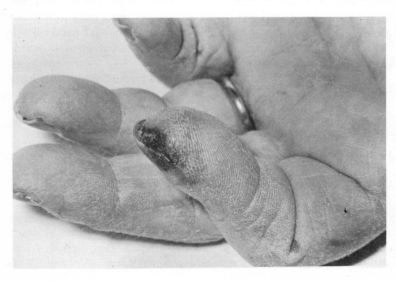

Involvement of blood vessels supplying the gut may result in an infarcted bowel with resultant gangrene, peritonitis and death. Treatment of arteritis is usually by high doses of prednisolone, by penicillamine or immuno-suppressive drugs. Simple nail fold lesions often respond to rest and absence of trauma.

Raynaud's phenomenon consists of pain and pallor in the hands when exposed to cold. It is a feature of rheumatoid disease and is associated with narrowing of the small arteries of the fingers caused by the arteritis.

Neuropathy

Rheumatoid arteritis is often associated with a neuropathy, ie a disorder of nerves. This may vary from mild interference with sensation causing numbness and pins and needles in the periphery to paralysis of motor nerves causing foot drop or wrist drop. When one or more large nerves are involved the condition is known as mononeuritis multiplex. Recovery from a neuropathy does occur but is often incomplete.

A common disorder of the nerves in rheumatoid arthritis is nerve entrapment. In certain body sites nerves run near structures which may compress them. The best known example is the carpal tunnel syndrome. Here the median nerve becomes compressed at the wrist where it runs into a tunnel formed from the flexor retinaculum and the bones of the carpus. Swelling of the synovium within this tunnel compresses the nerve. Typically the symptoms of pain in the hand and numbness of the thumb, index and middle fingers are worse at night and early morning. Other sites of nerve entrapment are the ulnar nerve at the elbow and the posterior tibial nerve at the ankle. Irritation of the ulnar nerve causes numbness and paraesthesia in the little and ring fingers and compression of the posterior tibial nerve causes similar symptoms in the feet. Treatment is simple but essential as continued nerve compression usually leads to muscle wasting and weakness as well as sensory loss. The usual methods of treatment of carpal tunnel syndrome are by corticosteroid injection into the carpal tunnel, by splinting or by surgical decompression.

Pericarditis

Pericarditis is inflammation of the sac which contains the heart. Pericarditis is found in 60% of rheumatoid patients at post-mortem, although in life it is rare for it to be detected clinically. Very occasionally pericarditis may result in severe fibrosis of the pericardium with constriction of the heart. Surgical release of the pericardium is needed to restore heart filling to normal.

Occasionally, rheumatoid inflammation or nodules may affect heart valves.

Respiratory complications

The respiratory complications of rheumatoid arthritis are pleural effusion, pulmonary fibrosis, rheumatoid nodules in the lung and Caplan's syndrome.

Pleural effusions are not uncommon and have to be differentiated from other causes such as infections and malignant effusions. Diagnostic aspiration is necessary for this.

Interstitial pulmonary fibrosis is detected normally on a routine radiograph. It is only rarely progressive and usually causes no symptoms perhaps because the patient's exercise tolerance is circumscribed by his arthritis.

Rheumatoid nodules in the lung may impose a diagnostic problem as on X-ray they may be indistinguishable from a tumour. Usually their character can be inferred but occasionally it is necessary to go to thoracotomy to establish the diagnosis.

Caplan's syndrome is found in miners with rheumatoid arthritis and consists of a particularly florid form of industrial lung dust disease (pneumoconiosis).

Sjogren's syndrome

Sjogren's syndrome is the combination of dry eyes, dry mouth and rheumatoid arthritis. The dry eyes and dry mouth are caused by inflammation of the lacrimal and salivary glands respectively. In mild degree this condition is very common in hospital patients with rheumatoid arthritis. A more severe form of the disease is known as the Sicca syndrome and is associated with failure of secretions in the bronchi, gut and vagina. Frequently in this condition the arthritis is only minor. Treatment in Sjogren's syndrome is symptomatic and by lubricant eye drops, and mouth washes.

Lymphadenopathy

Enlarged lymph glands are a feature of active rheumatoid arthritis in some patients. The glands can reach a large size and have to be differentiated from other causes of lymph gland enlargement. This may require biopsy.

Felty's syndrome

Felty's syndrome is a combination of rheumatoid arthritis and an enlarged spleen with features of what is known as hypersplenism. In this condition there are reduced numbers of platelets, white cells and red cells. Consequently the patient is anaemic, bruises easily and is liable to contract infection, and frequently has leg ulcers. Treatment is on the usual lines for rheumatoid arthritis, corticosteroids may improve the blood picture but sometimes splenectomy is necessary.

Eye complications

Apart from Sjogren's syndrome there are a number of complications which may affect the eye.

It may be in the form of inflammation of the white of the eye known as scleritis and occasionally patients present with red eyes. Frequent attacks of scleritis may result in the sclera producing a condition known as scleromalacia when the white of the eye has a blue to black appearance. Local treatment of scleritis is by corticosteroid eye drops.

Rheumatoid nodules may form in the sclera and if these nodules perforate, the contents of the eye may pass out through them and the condition is then known as scleritis perforans.

Amyloid disease

Amyloidosis is a condition in which a substance known as amyloid is laid down in various body tissues. The exact origin of the substance is unknown. In the most common form of the disease amyloidosis appears when there is any cause of continuing inflammation in the body, eg chronic osteomyelitis, bronchiectasis or rheumatoid arthritis. The condition is dangerous when it interferes with the function of vital tissues. In RA amyloid usually affects the kidneys. This is easily detected on ward testing and a rheumatoid patient with proteinuria should be suspected of having amyloidosis. Proteinuria may go on to a full nephrotic syndrome, chronic renal failure and death. Diagnosis is by biopsy. The usual sites for biopsy are the rectum (Fig. 3.16), gums or kidney. There is no definitive treatment

64

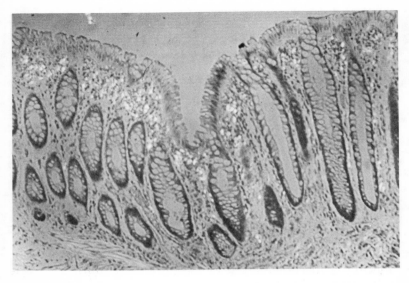

Fig. 3.16 Biopsy of rectal mucosa. The white specks are deposits of amyloid.

for it but every effort should be made to completely suppress disease activity.

Infections

In some patients with rheumatoid arthritis there is an increased susceptibility to infections. In these subjects recurrent spontaneous infections of joints occur. In normal people who develop an infected joint the joint is usually hot, swollen and very tender but in these patients with rheumatoid arthritis the joints may merely be painful and swollen. It is easy to mistake this for a flare-up of rheumatoid arthritis and it is important to remember the possibility of an infected joint in patients with chronic rheumatoid arthritis.

4

Juvenile Chronic Arthritis (Still's Disease, Juvenile Rheumatoid Arthritis)

Chronic arthritis in children is a relatively rare condition. A child can be said to have juvenile chronic arthritis when he has had arthritis for three months or more and the arthritis has been shown not to be due to other conditions which may cause arthritis or bone pain in children, eg infections of bones and joints, leukaemia and other malignancies, rheumatic fever, Henoch Schonlein purpura, sickle cell anaemia, etc (see list, p. 66). The diagnosis of juvenile chronic arthritis, therefore, rests heavily on the exclusion of other causes of arthritis. It may be necessary to perform a joint biopsy as well as blood tests and X-rays to confirm the diagnosis.

Juvenile chronic arthritis is sometimes called Still's disease after George Frederick Still who was one of the first to describe the condition.

In the United States, juvenile chronic arthritis is usually known as juvenile rheumatoid arthritis (JRA).

Prevalence

In the United Kingdom the prevalence is at least 6 per 10 000 of the school population. The peak age of incidence is from 1 to 5 years but babies can be affected within months of birth. Despite its rarity the condition is important as correct diagnosis and treatment are essential for the child's eventual well-being.

Juvenile Chronic Arthritis

Arthritis for more than 3 months
Patient aged less than 16 years
Other conditions, eg infection, malignancy, excluded
Type of Onset
  Systemic
  Polyarticular
  Oligo-articular

Some causes of bone pain and arthritis in children other than juvenile
chronic arthritis

Rheumatic fever
Henoch Schonlein purpura
Infections: Tuberculosis
               Salmonella
               Staphylococcal
               Viral, eg mumps, rubella
Malignancies: Leukaemia
               Reticulosarcoma
               Neuroblastoma
Legg-Perthes disease   ⎫
Slipped femoral epiphysis   ⎬   Causes of hip pain
Irritable hip syndrome   ⎭
Haemophilia
Sickle cell anaemia
Familial Mediterranean Fever
Dermatomyositis
Systemic sclerosis
Systemic lupus erythematosus

Clinical Features

There are three chief types of juvenile chronic arthritis or Still's
disease.

1. Systemic variety. In this condition the clinical picture is
dominated by fever, rash, splenomegaly, enlargement of glands and
sometimes pericarditis. The child may be very ill indeed and
systemic corticosteroids may be necessary to control the illness.
Arthritis though often present, need not be present at the start but
appears later.

2. Polyarticular type. In this type many joints are affected particularly the peripheral joints as in adult rheumatoid arthritis.

3. Oligo-articular type. This type exhibits arthritis in only one and
at the most a few joints and systemic disturbance is not marked.

However, 10% of children with this type of arthritis, especially girls, develop inflammation of iris of the eye (iritis or uveitis). This may eventually lead to blindness.

These three types are not exclusive and absolutely clear cut. In any one patient considerable overlap may occur. Some of these children will eventually turn out to have other forms of chronic arthritis such as psoriatic arthritis, ankylosing spondylitis or enteropathic arthritis. The family history may give a clue in these conditions as both psoriatic arthritis and spondylitis tend to be familial. In older children chronic arthritis may resemble adult arthritis from the start and present as, for example, sero-positive rheumatoid disease or ankylosing spondylitis.

Juvenile chronic arthritis differs from adult rheumatoid arthritis chiefly in the fact that the disease is in the setting of childhood with consequent developmental, social and educational impact. There are, however, a number of specific features peculiar to childhood arthritis:

(1) A tendency to joint ankylosis.
(2) An effect on growth. This applies both to local growth around an affected joint and applies to body growth in general.
(3) An effect on the eye, ie uveitis.

1. Prolonged immobilization easily leads to bony fusion and indeed this may take place without any enforced immobilization at all. This is clearly seen in the neck where the vertebral bodies may fuse into a solid block of bone (Fig. 4.1). Apart from bony fusion there is also a marked tendency to joint contractures if exercise is not regularly carried out.

2. Any chronic disease can affect a child's growth and Still's disease is no exception. However, they may catch up during remission and puberty, although delayed, does eventually occur. The effect of the disease on growth is made worse if corticosteroids are used in treatment. These drugs suppress growth hormone. The anti-growth effect is ameliorated if they are given on alternate days instead of daily. If steroids are stopped the child's growth tends to catch up. Clearly the small stature and delayed puberty causes anxiety when a patient compares himself to his fellows.

Local growth abnormalities occur around affected joints. Early fusion of epiphyses results in a shorter limb or digit and reduced growth of the mandible leads to the typical receding chin (micro-

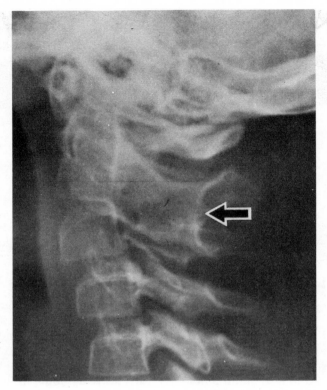

Fig. 4.1 The vertebral arches of the second and third cervical vertebrae are fused (arrow).

gnathia). Conversely, sometimes arthritis of a joint causes increased growth around it, so that the limb may in fact be longer than its fellow.

3. Inflammation of the ciliary body of the eye (iridocyclitis) occurs in 10% of patients with oligo–articular disease. The iris becomes adherent to the lens, cataract formation may occur and eventually glaucoma. The important feature in this condition is that in the young child it appears to be asymptomatic. The first indication of the disease may be severe loss of vision. The eyes often appear normal on inspection and special examination with a split lamp is needed to diagnose iritis and follow cases adequately (Fig. 4.2). This condition is more common in girls with anti–nuclear antibodies in the blood.

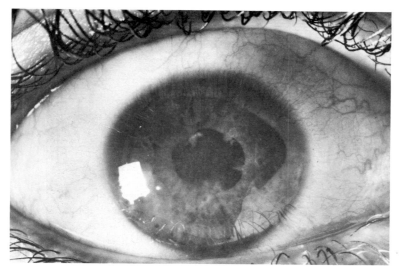

Fig. 4.2 Iritis in Still's disease. Note the irregular pupil and adhesions to the lens.
Photograph courtesy of Dr. Barbara M. Ansell

An acute and less damaging form of iritis occurs in boys with ankylosing spondylitis.

Laboratory investigations

During the acute phases of the disease there is often an anaemia and the ESR is high. The rheumatoid factor is usually absent from the blood but anti-nuclear antibody may be present. There is an increased chance of eye complications in children with positive anti-nuclear antibody. Immunoglobulins should always be measured as agammaglobulinaemia is an uncommon cause of juvenile arthritis. Height and weight should be routinely measured and recorded on a percentile chart.

Management

Drugs. The object of treatment is to relieve pain, reduce joint swelling and tenderness and lower the pyrexia if there is one. Aspirin is given in doses of 90 to 150 mg per kg/body weight. Blood salicylate level should be measured and a level of about 25 mg per 100 ml should be aimed for. Salicylate intoxication in young children should be watched for. It consists of over breathing, dehydration and psychological disturbances such as confusion and out-of-character behaviour.

```
┌────────────────────────────────────────────────┐
│                                                  │
│   Effect of aspirin overdose in young children   │
│                                                  │
│            1. Unusual behaviour                  │
│            2. Over breathing                     │
│            3. Dehydration                        │
│          . 4. Bleeding                           │
│                                                  │
└────────────────────────────────────────────────┘
```

Alternatives to soluble aspirin are benorylate, ibuprofen and indomethacin. These can all be given in liquid form.

Gold or penicillamine may also be used in Still's disease to induce a remission if the condition is unresponsive to these prior measures. The doses are smaller and depend on the child's size. The side effects are similar to the adult. Chloroquine may be fatally poisonous to young children in small doses (about one gram) and is consequently little used. The antigrowth disadvantage of corticosteroids adds to their other side effects in children but they are sometimes necessary to control very active systemic disease. If possible alternate day therapy should be instituted as this decreases the side effects of corticosteroids. Drugs such as azathioprine, cyclophosphamide and chlorambucil have been used in resistant cases of juvenile chronic arthritis particularly in those complicated by amyloidosis.

Splinting. Rest splints made of plaster of Paris are used to maintain joints in the correct position during sleep and after exercises particularly around the wrists and knees. Serial splinting may sometimes be necessary to reduce contractures and light plastic work splints to support a joint and relieve pain enable a particular function to be carried out, eg writing. A light plastic collar is used to prevent neck flexion deformities. The feet should be supported by long arch supports or in well-fitting shoes.

Rest. Rest is used sparingly in children because of the tendency for osteoporosis, joint contractures and premature fusion of the epiphyses to take place. However, a child should be encouraged not to bear weight on a painful joint and bed rest is necessary in the acute systemic variety of the disease. When the child is resting in bed it is essential that the joints are kept mobile and rested in the correct position. Painful hips will sometimes respond to a combination of bed rest and traction. Regular prone lying should be performed daily to prevent and correct hip contractures (Fig. 4.3).

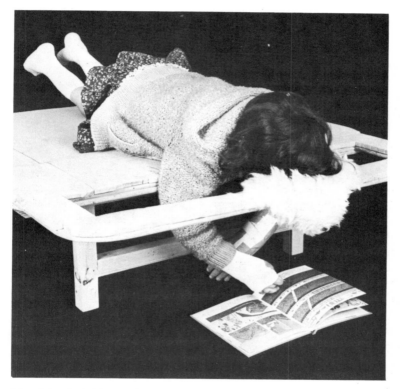

Fig. 4.3 A child with flexion contractures of the hips using a prone lying couch.

Exercises. Exercises are necessary to treat and prevent contractures and strengthen weak muscles. Exercises should be made as much a part of daily activities and play as possible. The ward staff have an active role in carrying out exercises set by the physiotherapist. At home it is the chief responsibility of the parents to ensure that these exercises take place. Hydrotherapy in a warm pool plays an important part in maintaining good musculature and joint movement without the trauma of weight bearing and for this reason it is especially useful in childhood arthritis. It is also fun. Activities such as cycling and swimming which exercise the joints without weight bearing should be encouraged.

Surgery. Surgery is less applicable in chronic childhood arthritis than in the adult. It may be important in establishing the diagnosis through synovial biopsy. Synovectomy of the knee may be carried

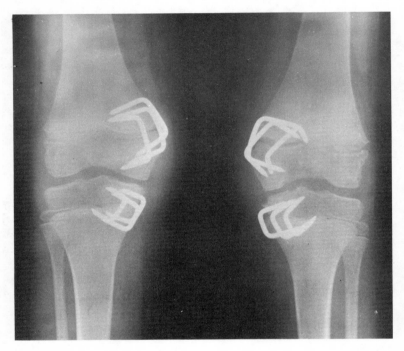

Fig. 4.4 The X-ray shows metal staples inserted to correct epiphyseal growth.

out for the persistent synovitis unresponsive to other forms of treatment. Procedures to correct deformity such as stapling of the epiphyses of the knee (Fig. 4.4) or osteotomy to correct valgus deformities may be necessary. Hip replacement can be performed in teenagers.

Education. The education of children is especially important as they will have to earn their living by intellectual rather than by physical means. Their education may be in a hospital school, in a special school for the disabled, from a visiting teacher or in a normal school. The latter though preferable and possible in a small primary school, is more difficult in a large secondary school as much unsupervised travel has to take place between classrooms. Children will need guidance on careers and reassurance and advice about their ability to fulfil adult roles including those of marriage, child bearing and child rearing.

Family involvement. It is essential that a child's family be made aware of all aspects of treatment. Parents must have some understanding of the rationale of therapy and should be capable of and encouraged to do simple physiotherapy at home. Nursing staff are sometimes more available than doctors to answer queries from parents. Case conferences at crucial periods in the child's progress are especially valuable and should include all interested parties such as teachers, employment officers and social workers as well as of course the parents and child.

Prognosis

The outlook in general is good. Over 80% of children eventually survive to become independent adults albeit sometimes with residual deformities. A few die from the disease mainly from renal amyloidosis and infection. The remainder become severely crippled or perhaps blind. However, the proportion doing well is still greater than that in patients with adult rheumatoid arthritis attending hospital and it is justifiable to take a generally optimistic attitude when dealing with parents and relatives.

Further reading

Allin, R. E. and Lawton, D. S. *The Management of Juvenile Chronic Polyarthritis*. Association of Paediatric Chartered Physiotherapists. (Obtainable from the Physiotherapy Department, Brays School, Brays Road, Birmingham, B26 1NS.)

Ansell, Barbara M. *Rheumatic Disorders in Childhood*. In series *Clinics in Rheumatic Diseases*. W. B. Saunders & Co. Ltd.

Bywaters, E. G. L., 'The Management of Juvenile Chronic Polyarthritis', *Bulletin on the Rheumatic Diseases*, vol. 27, no. 2, p. 882.

5
Sero–negative Arthritis

The term sero–negative arthritis covers a group of diseases which have certain features in common. They comprise the following clinical entities: idiopathic ankylosing spondylitis, psoriatic arthritis, Reiter's disease and enteropathic arthritis.

These diseases are characterized by the absence of rheumatoid factor in the blood, hence the term sero–negative. In addition the following features are common to all or some of the conditions.

(1) A tendency to involve the larger and medium sized joints.
(2) Arthritis of the sacro–iliac joints (sacroiliitis) and an inflammatory arthritis of the joints of the spine (spondylitis).
(3) Inflammation of the eye.
(4) Urethritis.
(5) Skin rash.
(6) Inflammation of the aorta where it arises from the heart (aortitis).
(7) An increased prevalence of the tissue type HLA B27.

Sero–negative arthritis
(sero–negative spondyloarthritis)

1. Idiopathic ankylosing spondylitis
2. Psoriatic arthritis
3. Reiter's disease
4. Enteropathic arthritis

Idiopathic ankylosing spondylitis

Ankylosing spondylitis is a condition in which an inflammatory arthritis affects the sacro–iliac and spinal joints eventually resulting in bone fusion (ankylosis).

Prevalence and epidemiology

Ankylosing spondylitis is a common condition occurring more commonly in males than females, with a ratio of 4 to 1. The prevalence is about 5 per 1000 males but this may be an underestimate and the disease may be as common as 1 per 100 of the general population. The disease is very rare in negroes.

Aetiology

The precise cause of ankylosing spondylitis is unknown but there is a strong familial and inherited tendency. The relatives of a spondylitic have an approximate 20-fold increased chance of acquiring the condition. This makes the incidence of the disease very high in some inbred communities, eg the Haidu Indians of Vancouver Island have a prevalence of 6.1% of the population. The genetic component of the disease is illustrated by the fact that 95% of ankylosing spondylitics have the tissue type HLA B27.

Pathology

The condition usually affects the sacro-iliac joints causing inflammation and erosion of the joint margins. After some time this inflammation dies down and the joints are replaced by bone obliterating and ankylosing them.

In the spine both the intervertebral disc joints and synovial apophyseal joints are involved. Inflammatory changes at the junction of disc and vertebrae are followed by extensive ossification of the outer layers of the disc, joining vertebral bodies together by a rigid sheet of bone. The interior of the discs is replaced by fibrous tissue. Similar changes take place in the apophyseal joints so that eventually the whole spine from coccyx to skull may become a rigid pole of bone (Fig. 5.1).

An inflammatory peripheral arthritis indistinguishable histologically from rheumatoid arthritis occurs in a proportion of spondylitics. Sixty-four per cent of spondylitics have hip, shoulder or peripheral joint involvement. Up to 25% of cases develop inflammation of the eye, usually iritis, and about 3% develop cardiac complications, the number increasing as the years go by to about 10% at 30 years' duration of illness. The cardiac complications consist of dilatation of the aortic ring and interference with conduction in the heart. Urethritis is also more common in ankylosing spondylitis and other

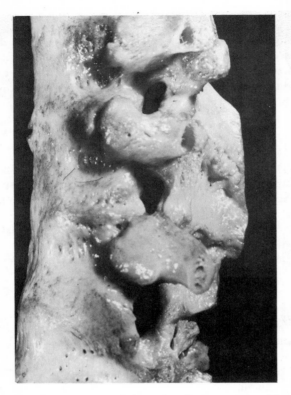

Fig. 5.1 This shows part of the spine from a man with ankylosing spondylitis. There is complete bony ankylosis of all the spinal joints.

complications include amyloidosis, pulmonary fibrosis in the apices of the lungs and interferences with nerve roots in the lumbar spine.

Clinical features

The patients are usually young men. The presenting complaint is of low back pain, sciatica or chest pain and the pains are frequently associated with morning stiffness. In the active phase of the disease the pain may be very severe. Examination reveals a stiff back with restricted chest movements (Fig. 5.2). About 20% present with a peripheral arthritis and this is especially true of women. Fatigue is a pronounced feature of ankylosing spondylitis.

In some individuals the condition is remarkable by the lack of

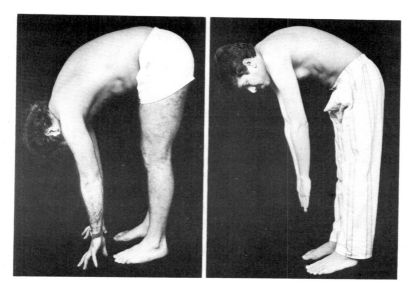

Fig. 5.2 (a) normal back movement; (b) the stiff lumbar spine and early dorsal kyphosis of spondylitis.

symptoms and it may then only be diagnosed from a radiographic examination made for another purpose.

Course and prognosis

The course of the disease is usually progressive. The tendency is for pain and stiffness to move from the lumbar area to the neck and the limb girdles. The spine loses its normal lumbar lordosis and the normal dorsal kyphosis becomes exaggerated. This means that the patient is only able to look forward by craning the neck back. If the cervical spine becomes fixed as well then the patient is unable to look forward at all when walking or to correct his stoop. The disability of a rigid spine is made very much worse by stiffening and reduction in the range of movement of the hip joints. In some people the disease appears to go into spontaneous remission.

Complications of ankylosing spondylitis are a cause of death in about 10% of cases, usually due to renal amyloidosis or heart disease. For the majority of sufferers the functional prognosis is good, most remaining active and in employment.

Treatment

The pain of ankylosing spondylitis responds well to such drugs as phenylbutazone (100 mg 2–3 times a day), indomethacin (25 mg four times a day) and naproxen (250 mg twice a day). These drugs will have to be continued for most of the patient's life apart from natural remissions. For particularly severe cases, short courses of local deep X-ray therapy to the spine may relieve pain for many months. There is however an increased risk of developing leukaemia after these radiotherapy treatments, although the interval between the onset of the leukaemia and the radiotherapy may be many years.

Exercises to avoid the spondylitic spinal deformities are essential. These exercises are basically back extension exercises. They should be taught firstly in a physiotherapy department and the patient then encouraged to do them at home (see Appendix A, p. 220).

Regular follow-up is needed to check that the exercise programme is being complied with and to examine patients regularly for complications. Spondylitics are often very active but pain and fatigue may be very debilitating causing them to require considerable psychological support from time to time. It is important to emphasize the good functional prognosis for most spondylitics.

Complications such as iritis and heart disease need expert attention from the appropriate specialist. Heart valve replacement and cardiac pacing may be necessary.

Surgery

Surgery has two main applications in ankylosing spondylitis. The most common is hip replacement. A stiff back makes mobile hips essential. The perfection of the hip arthroplasty has been of immense benefit to many patients with ankylosing spondylitis. The operation is performed in the usual way although in some centres there has been a tendency for the hips to stiffen up after the operation but this is not the universal experience.

Spinal osteotomy is sometimes necessary. This is used in a patient with a rigid curved spine and is performed in order to improve posture. It is a difficult operation to perform and damage to the spinal cord and nerves is a possibility. It may enable a patient to face forwards instead of forever staring at the ground.

Assessment

The assessment and advice of an occupational therapist is valuable in the spondylitics especially those who develop restriction of hip movement.

Reiter's disease

Hans Reiter, a German army doctor, described the syndrome of arthritis, urethritis and conjunctivitis occurring after dysentery in German troops in Salonica in the First World War. This combination of symptoms has since been called Reiter's syndrome or disease. The disease is now more commonly seen following a non-gonococcal urethritis (non-specific urethritis). It is frequently accompanied by other features as shown below.

Reiter's disease

1. Non-specific urethritis
2. Arthritis
3. Conjunctivitis or uritis
4. Oral and penile ulcers
5. Keratoderma blennorrhagica
6. Predominantly a disease of young men

Aetiology

Reiter's disease is a reaction to infection. In the post-dysenteric type, the infection is caused by bacteria such as Shigella and Yersinia. In non-specific urethritis an organism known as Chlamydia has been isolated from the urethral discharge of some patients. These organisms are intermediate between viruses and bacteria. Treatment with antibiotics does not seem to affect the course of Reiter's disease.

There is no doubt that Reiter's disease occurs in those constitutionally inclined to develop it. Only about 1% of men who contract non-gonococcal urethritis develop Reiter's disease. Seventy-six per cent of men acquiring Reiter's disease have HLA B27 tissue type or to put it another way, a man who contracts urethritis and has a B27 tissue type has forty times the chance of developing Reiter's disease compared to another man with urethritis and without B27.

Clinical features

Following urethritis, conjunctivitis is usually the first manifestation followed by the arthritis.

The urethral discharge is sterile and may be complicated by prostatitis. Occasionally the urethral discharge may not be apparent but

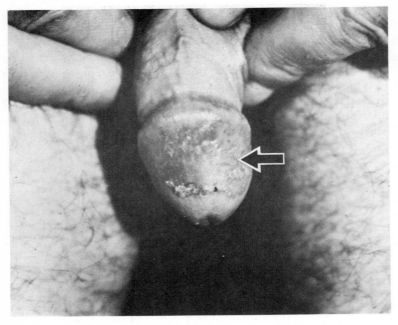

Fig. 5.3 Balanitis in Reiter's disease. Arrow points to ulcers.

may present as dysuria. The conjunctivitis is usually transient but iritis (uveitis) may occur.

The arthritis typically attacks a few large joints but the joints of the feet are also frequently involved. Painful heels are a feature of Reiter's disease. Sacro-iliac joints are often involved but this may be only apparent on X-ray. Aspiration of joints reveals that synovial fluid which is frequently pus-like in character is sterile on culture.

Ulcers in the mouth occur and are usually painless and the patient is unaware of them. Ulcers around the glans penis may coalesce to form a circinate balanitis (Fig. 5.3). Occasionally this balanitis may be frankly purulent and again the discharge is sterile.

The skin disease is characteristic and the last of the manifestations to occur. Pustules full of keratin form on the soles of the feet forming a patchy white sheet over the sole (Fig. 5.4). They look very unsightly but eventually the hyperkeratotic rash falls off to leave unmarked and normal skin. A similar process under the nails lifts them off the nail bed and distorts them (Fig. 5.5). Again the affected nails eventually separate and fall away leaving normal tissue behind.

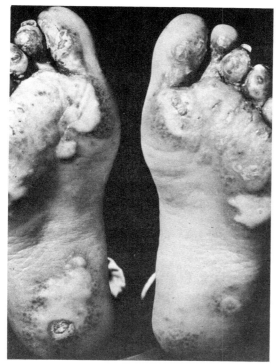

Fig. 5.4 Keratoderma blennoraghica in Reiter's disease.
Fig. 5.5 The nails in Reiter's disease.

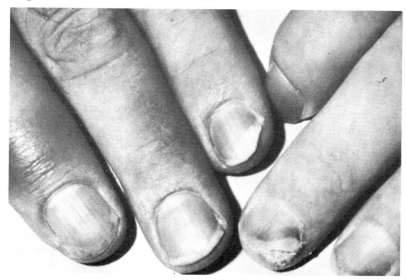

The appearance of the nails in Reiter's disease is very similar to that in psoriasis.

Laboratory investigations

The ESR is raised during the acute phase of the disease and tests for rheumatoid factor and other auto-antibodies are negative. X-rays may show a periostitis in the early stages and later show erosions around affected joints.

Treatment

Treatment is on the general lines for acute arthritis. Indomethacin and phenylbutazone will largely control pain and stiffness. Local aspiration of the joints and steroid injections into joints may be necessary. Splinting and reduced weight bearing are sometimes required to control symptoms. In very severe cases it may be necessary to treat with systemic steroids or cytotoxic drugs such as methotrexate or azathioprine.

In severe cases, this is a most unpleasant illness and skilled nursing with adequate genital toilet and local care for the skin lesions are essential to make life bearable.

Prognosis and course of the disease

In most cases recovery takes place within two to sixteen weeks of the illness starting but sometimes full recovery may take well up to a year in severe cases and the course may be marked by exacerbations and remissions.

The long-term prognosis is less certain. In one series reviewed, twenty years after the initial illness, no less than 32% had developed spondylitis, 18% had developed a chronic peripheral arthritis and 7% had developed uveitis.

As in ankylosing spondylitis a few cases develop heart disease, mainly aortitis.

Psoriatic Arthritis

Psoriasis is a common skin disease and arthritis is more common amongst psoriatic sufferers than in the population as a whole. About 6.8% of psoriatic patients have an inflammatory arthritis. People with psoriasis may suffer from rheumatoid arthritis and osteoarthritis like anyone else but there are types of arthritis especially associated with psoriasis.

Types of psoriatic arthritis

1. Distal interphalangeal joint arthritis
2. Asymmetrical polyarthritis
3. Sero-negative rheumatoid arthritis
4. Arthritis mutilans
5. Sacroiliitis and spondylitis

Aetiology

The cause of psoriatic arthritis is unknown. Heredity plays a large part. It is common to find relatives with psoriatic arthritis and in fact, psoriatic arthritis runs in families as does psoriasis. Relatives of a patient with psoriatic arthritis have a fifty-fold chance of developing the condition. There seem to be two sorts of family, those with both psoriasis and arthritis and those with just psoriasis alone.

The relationship of psoriasis to the arthritis is not constant. The psoriasis may precede, accompany or postdate the onset of the arthritis. In families the different manifestations of psoriasis and arthritis may present separately in different individuals. One may have one relative with psoriasis, one with a peripheral arthritis without psoriasis and another with spondylitis. It is clear that psoriatic arthritis in an individual may occur, therefore, without demonstrable psoriasis and in these cases the only way to make a definite diagnosis is to obtain a good family history. As in other sero-negative arthritides, HLA B27 is more common both in those with sacroiliitis and spondylitis and also in those with peripheral arthritis.

The precipitating cause of arthritis in a particular joint is not known. However, the theory of the deep Koebner phenomenon attempts to explain it. In a patient with psoriasis, trauma to the skin often produces a patch of psoriasis along the line of the trauma. The deep Koebner phenomenon theory suggests that trauma to an individual joint somehow produces a psoriatic reaction within that joint.

Under the microscope the synovial changes are similar to rheumatoid arthritis.

Clinical features

On the whole the male to female ratio is about 1:1 except in sero-negative rheumatoid arthritis where the usual female predominance applies.

1. Distal interphalangeal joint arthritis is especially associated with psoriasis. It often affects fingers in which the nail is also severely affected by psoriasis.

2. Other finger joints may be involved and if so are affected in a random and asymmetrical way. The joint swelling is often more diffuse than in rheumatoid arthritis and the skin may be red. In the feet this diffuse swelling often involves the whole digit producing sausage toes (psoriatic dactylitis, Fig. 5.6).

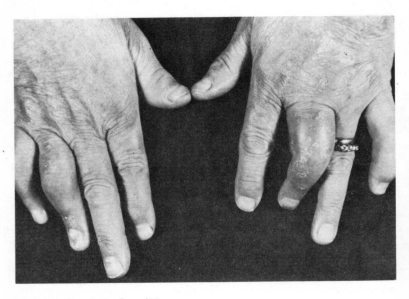

Fig. 5.6 Psoriatic dactylitis.

It is common for one or two medium or large joints to be affected with psoriatic arthritis and these joints may become grossly inflamed with considerable pain, swelling and tenderness and even fever. Aspiration of the joint reveals sterile pus. When the onset is acute it closely resembles gout.

3. Sero-negative rheumatoid arthritis. This condition resembles

rheumatoid arthritis in every way except that rheumatoid factor is absent and the disease is, therefore, referred to as being sero-negative.

4. Arthritis mutilans. This condition affects a very small proportion of people with psoriatic arthritis. They usually have severe cutaneous psoriasis. There is widespread destruction of joints with multiple dislocations leading to flail hands and wrists and very severe disability (Fig. 5.7).

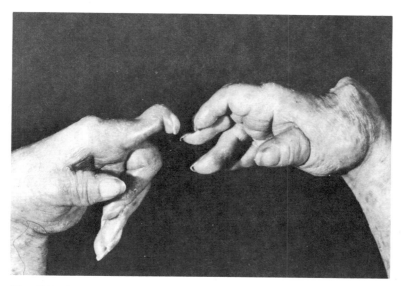

Fig. 5.7 Psoriatic arthritis mutilans. Note extensive cutaneous psoriasis and joint dislocations.

5. Sacroiliitis and spondylitis. Sacroiliitis occurs in 20% of patients with psoriasis. Spondylitis occurs in a slightly smaller proportion. The symptoms of back pain and stiffness are the same as in ankylosing spondylitis and similar complications may occur.

X-ray features

Some features of psoriatic arthritis produce characteristic X-ray pictures. Severe destruction of bone may be seen on X-ray (osteolysis) often with little or no osteoporosis. Sometimes whittling of a phalanx may occur with spreading of the more distal phalanx producing a pencil-in-cup deformity. Other X-ray changes are similar to those seen in rheumatoid arthritis and/or ankylosing spondylitis.

Laboratory

In the active phase, the ESR is raised and there may be an anaemia. Tests for rheumatoid factor are negative. Examination of synovial fluid reveals many white cells but culture for organisms is negative. The serum uric acid may be raised in psoriasis.

Treatment

Treatment is on similar lines to rheumatoid arthritis and spondylitis. However, one must bear in mind that in the vast majority of cases the prognosis is better than in rheumatoid arthritis and therefore the use of dangerous drugs is less justified. Drugs may also exacerbate the psoriasis. This is particularly true of chloroquine and probably gold and penicillamine. Nurses in gold clinics and those dealing with psoriatic patients who are on such drugs should be particularly aware that any flare-up of their psoriasis may be due to drugs. Patients with severe cutaneous psoriasis have a marked social handicap. Marital breakdown is common. Treatment, therefore, should be directed as much against the skin as against the joint disease although treating the skin does not produce a remission in the arthritis.

Prognosis

The prognosis is good on the whole in psoriatic arthritis, especially in those people with TIP involvement and sero-negative rheumatoid arthritis. Not surprisingly those patients with arthritis mutilans do much worse than these two groups but fortunately this is a relatively rare manifestation of the disease.

Patients as a rule tend to suffer intermittent bouts of arthritis which leave no mark or one or two joints stiffened.

Enteropathic Arthritis

This collective term is used to describe arthritides which are associated with bowel disease.

Gut Diseases associated with Arthritis
1. Ulcerative colitis
2. Crohn's disease or regional ileitis
3. Infective enteritis
4. Gut resection
5. Whipple's disease

Colitic arthritis. An arthritis occurs in 11% of patients with ulcerative colitis. The arthritis chiefly involves the large joints of the lower limbs and is not destructive. It is associated particularly with severe and widespread bowel disease and exacerbated synchronously with the colitis. Removal of the bowel (proctocolectomy) results in a remission of the arthritis. Two per cent of colitic patients also have or develop ankylosing spondylitis. In contrast to the peripheral arthritis this progresses without relation to exacerbation of colitis or to removal of the diseased bowel.

Treatment is on the general lines for an inflammatory arthritis with a proviso that the prognosis for the joints is good. These patients are also more likely to lose blood from the bowel with anti-inflammatory drugs like aspirin or indomethacin. Hand deformities may make handling of ileostomy appliances difficult. Ankylosing spondylitis is managed on the regimen for ankylosing spondylitis.

Arthritis of Crohn's disease. Crohn's disease or regional ileitis is less common than ulcerative colitis. It may also be associated with a similar peripheral arthritis and with ankylosing spondylitis particularly if the disease involves the large bowel. Approximately 20% of patients with Crohn's disease have peripheral arthritis and 2% have ankylosing spondylitis.

Postenteric arthritis. Certain gastrointestinal infections may be associated with an arthritis, the best known being postenteric arthritis which may follow gut infections with salmonella. The inflamed joints are sterile and the arthritis which eventually resolves without serious joint damage seems to be a reaction to the infection.

Arthritis associated with gastrointestinal bypass surgery. In some centres obesity is treated by 'short circuiting' part of the intestine surgically. In a few cases this has resulted in an arthritis.

Whipple's disease. This is a potentially fatal disease of middle-aged men. It consists of steatorrhoea and arthritis although ankylosing spondylitis is also an occasional complication. The cause was for a long time unknown but recently organisms have been found in the gut and the joints, and the condition does respond to antibiotics.

6
Crystal Arthritis

Crystal arthritis is a collective term to describe those types of arthritis where symptoms are due to the presence within the joint of crystals; it is probably the irritant mechanical properties of the crystals that gives rise to symptoms as well as their chemical composition. Gout has been known for many years but more recently another type of arthritis, which clinically resembles gout, has been recognized and is known as pseudogout.

Gout

Gout is an inflammatory arthritis, due to the deposition of urate crystals within a joint.

Aetiology

Uric acid is normally dissolved in solution and is present in most body fluids, including synovial fluid, as sodium urate. With raised levels, depending partly on the acidity of the tissues, the urate crystallizes out of the solution. If this occurs in a joint then an attack of gout results.

Uric acid is the end product in the breakdown of purines, which are themselves derived from the breakdown of nucleoproteins which come from cell nuclei. The last two stages in this process are important in the treatment of gout.

$$\text{Hypoxanthine} \longrightarrow \text{xanthine} \longrightarrow \text{uric acid}$$

An enzyme, xanthine oxidase, controls both of these final stages in the breakdown of purines.

The serum uric acid level reflects the balance between the production of uric acid and its excretion via the kidneys and the gut. The kidney is the major organ of excretion, only about 30% being excreted via the gut. Serum levels will be raised, therefore, if there is an increased formation of uric acid or a decreased excretion (Fig. 6.1).

Gout
1. Primary
2. Secondary

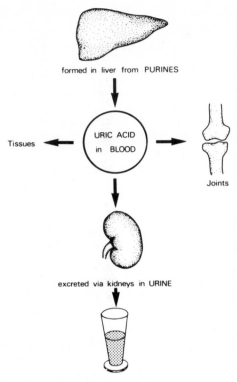

formed in liver from PURINES

Tissues ← URIC ACID in BLOOD → Joints

excreted via kidneys in URINE

Fig. 6.1 Pathways of uric acid metabolism.

Over-production occurs when there is an excessive breakdown of cells, for example, in blood diseases such as leukaemia and polycythemia. Dietary intake has only a small effect on serum uric acid levels. Reduced excretion will occur in any type of renal failure. Certain diuretics (thiazides, frusemide and ethacrynic acid) also reduce the renal excretion of uric acid. Aspirin in small doses blocks the excretion of uric acid, but in high doses (several grams a day) increases the amount excreted.

Both these causes of over-production and reduced excretion are sometimes called 'secondary' gout, ie the gout is secondary to an obvious abnormality. In most cases of gout none of these causes are present and such cases are known as 'primary', to distinguish them from the secondary cases mentioned above. In primary gout there is often a family history of gout in a blood relative. Primary gout may come about by an inborn error of metabolism, that either causes an increased production of uric acid or reduces the excretion, or may be a combination of these factors.

```
Causes of Secondary Gout

1. Over-production
     Blood diseases
2. Reduced excretion in urine
     Renal failure
     Certain diuretics
     Aspirin (in small doses)
```

Pathology

Uric acid crystals form more easily in an acid fluid and crystallization tends to occur in tissues with a poor blood supply, the pinna of the ear, joint cartilage and tendons. In the joint the result is an acute attack of gout. At other sites, if the collection of crystals becomes sizeable, it is called a tophus (pl. tophi). Persistent deposition in the cartilage of joints leads to degeneration of the cartilage and formation in the bone ends of cysts full of urate crystals; eventually a secondary osteoarthrosis develops. Large tophi near to the skin may break down and discharge urate crystals through a sinus. Crystals forming in the pelvis of the kidney may lead to renal stones. Occasionally a tophus is present in the kidney itself. Some degree of renal failure is common in long-standing untreated gout but usually the kidneys are scarred by fibrosis without any tophi being present. About 10% of people with primary gout also have high blood pressure.

```
Complications of Gout

1. Degeneration of cartilage and
     secondary osteoarthrosis
2. Tophi
3. Renal stones
4. Renal failure
```

Clinical Features

Gout rarely occurs in men before puberty and in women until after the menopause. The first attack is usually mono-articular and occurs in 80% of cases in the metatarso-phalangeal joint of the big toe. The onset of symptoms is usually acute with pain, tenderness and swelling of the affected joint and within a few hours the skin overlying the joint becomes warm and red. The pain may be exceptionally severe, so that the patient is unable to bear the weight of the bedclothes on the affected foot. There may be an associated fever and feeling of ill-health. Untreated the attack settles over seven to fourteen days.

There is then usually an interval of weeks, maybe months and occasionally years, before the next attack. Recurrent attacks then tend to occur at shorter intervals and other joints become affected, occasionally at the same time, producing a polyarticular disease. Tophi begin to appear and the term 'chronic tophaceous gout' is now applied.

Clinical Features

1. Mono–articular and onset in 80% of cases in big toe
2. Acute onset
3. Severe pain with redness of the skin overlying the joint
4. Untreated, settles 7–14 days

Investigations

The most important investigation is to demonstrate the presence of urate crystals in the synovial fluid during an attack or the presence of such crystals in a tophus. The finding of a high serum uric acid level is supporting evidence but is not diagnostic. During an acute attack the white blood count is usually raised, as is the ESR. Other investigations done at this time will be a full blood count and blood urea to exclude any seconday causes of gout. An X-ray of the affected joint

---

Investigations

1. Aspiration of joint
2. Aspiration of a tophus
3. Serum uric acid and blood urea
4. Full blood count and ESR
5. X-ray of joint

early in the disease will be normal but after repeated attacks a large cystic area in the bone adjacent to the joint may be seen. Urate crystals are not visible on X-ray. Eventually a secondary osteo-arthrosis will develop with more damage to the joint.

Treatment

Treatment is divided into two parts: (1) treatment of the acute attack, and (2) treatment to prevent further attacks.

The acute attack is treated by rest of the involved joint; usually the pain is so severe anyway that the patient is very unwilling to move the joint. The main drugs used to treat the attack are colchicine, phenylbutazone and indomethacin.

Colchicine is the oldest preparation but is slow to act and the effective dose is near to the toxic dose. Nowadays it is little used for treatment of the acute attack. Phenylbutazone is a very effective drug, given in a dose of 600 mg to start with and then 200 mg 6 hourly for 24 hours, and thereafter 200 mg tds, until the symptoms settle, usually within 48 hours. Indomethacin has a similar effect to phenylbutazone. *Note:* aspirin should never be used as in low dosage it blocks the excretion of uric acid and thus may make an attack worse.

Further attacks can be prevented by drugs which lower the serum uric acid level. The problem is when to start this treatment, for it has to be continued for life. Certainly it should not be given until the diagnosis is established beyond all doubt. It should probably not be started until attacks are occurring fairly frequently and the patient is prepared to prevent these by taking daily therapy for the rest of his life.

Remembering that the serum uric acid level reflects the balance between formation and excretion, it will be seen that the level can be lowered by either reducing formation or increasing excretion.

Drugs which increase the amount excreted in the urine are called uricosuric drugs; probenecid and sulphinpyrazone act in this way. Any reduction in the serum level of uric acid may initially be accompanied by more frequent attacks of gout. The patient needs to be warned of this when treatment is started otherwise he will think that the treatment is making his condition worse. The frequency of these attacks can perhaps be reduced by giving a daily dose of colchicine. Uricosuric drugs, because they increase the amount of urate in the urine, may be associated with the development of renal stones and to prevent this a large fluid intake should be encouraged and the urine kept alkaline by taking sodium bicarbonate. Uricosuric drugs are not effective in the presence of renal failure.

Allopurinol works by reducing the formation of uric acid. It inhibits the enzyme xanthine oxidase which is essential for the last two stages in the formation of uric acid (hypoxanthine⟶ xanthine⟶uric acid). Purines are therefore excreted as xanthine and hypoxanthine. These are more soluble than uric acid and so do not form crystals, nor give rise to renal stones. Allopurinol is effective in renal failure. Colchicine may be given in addition in a small daily dose in the hope of reducing any attacks over the first three to six months of treatment. Treatment will need to be continued for life. So far as we know at present there are no serious side effects from this treatment and Allopurinol is probably now the drug of choice, to prevent further attacks of gout.

Treatment of Gout

1. *Acute attack*
   Colchicine
   Phenylbutazone
   Indomethacin
2. *Prevention*
   Probenecid   ⎱ with or
   Sulphinpyrazone   ⎬ without
   Allopurinol   ⎰ colchicine

Pseudogout

Pseudogout is due to the deposition within the joint of crystals of calcium pyrophosphate (CPP). The crystals may be deposited within the synovial fluid and/or the articular cartilage.

Clinical Features

The crystals, if deposited in the synovial fluid, act in a very similar manner to urate crystals and produce an acute inflammatory arthritis, very similar to gout, hence the name pseudogout. The attacks tend to occur in middle age but unlike gout, rarely in the big toe and are more common in the large joints, particularly the knees. The clinical picture is of a sudden onset of arthritis with severe pain, swelling and tenderness of the joints. Sometimes, as in gout, there is an associated systemic illness with fever and malaise. Without treatment the attack settles in seven to ten days time. When the fluid is aspirated no urate crystals are found; instead there will be crystals of calcium pyrophosphate. These can be distinguished in the laboratory from urate crystals by using a polarizing microscope.

Pseudogout

1. Acute attacks due to the deposition of calcium pyrophosphate in synovial fluid
2. Calcium pyrophosphate deposited in articular cartilage leads to visible calcification on X-ray (chondrocalcinosis)

If the crystals are deposited within the joint cartilage then calcification of the cartilage appears on X-ray and this appearance is known as chondrocalcinosis. The relationship of calcification within the articular cartilage to arthritis is uncertain. Mild calcification, particularly in the knees, is common in older people and may be symptomless. Widespread calcification in articular cartilage is less common. It may also be symptomless or it may be associated with acute attacks of pseudogout. In some cases it may be associated with widespread degenerative disease of the joint. This uncertain relationship between the X-ray appearance and symptoms and subsequent disease is still being evaluated. Occasionally chondrocalcinosis is associated with hyperparathyroidism or haemachromatosis; however, most cases seem to be idiopathic and are not related to any gross disorder of calcium metabolism.

Clinical Features of Pseudogout

1. Sudden inflammation in joints, similar to gout
2. More common in larger joints
3. Rare in big toe

Treatment

The acute attack does not respond very well to colchicine but is treated otherwise like gout, with rest of the joint, indomethacin or phenylbutazone. In the larger joints aspiration of synovial fluid and injection of hydrocortisone is additionally helpful.

Chondrocalcinosis, where it is causing symptoms, is treated along similar lines to osteoarthrosis, with analgesic drugs, etc. There is no specific treatment to reduce the calcification.

7
Rheumatic Fever

Rheumatic fever follows infection with a particular type of streptococci (group A betahaemolytic streptococci), usually causing a
throat infection, and may affect the heart, joints, central nervous
system or skin. Its importance lies in the fact that it may cause
permanent damage to the heart.

Aetiology

Rheumatic fever is a disease of children and young adults. It is rare
before the age of five and after the age of eighteen and most cases
occur about the age of seven. Streptococcal throat infections are
common but only in about ½% of such infections does rheumatic
fever develop. There must, therefore, be other factors which influence its development but we are ignorant of what these factors may
be. Certainly rheumatic fever is not due to the direct action of the
streptococci on the heart. It is probable that antibodies produced as a
response to the streptococcal infection also attack the heart. Rheumatic fever is now much less common than it used to be.

Features of Rheumatic Fever

1. Follows group A betahaemolytic streptococcal
   infection
2. Fever
3. Arthritis
4. Carditis
5. Chorea
6. Nodules
7. Erythema marginatum

Clinical features

Rheumatic fever follows one to six weeks after the streptococcal
infection, with an average delay of three weeks. The clinical features
of rheumatic fever consist of fever, arthritis, carditis, chorea, sub-
cutaneous nodules and erythema marginatum.

Fever. Fever occurs in all cases of active rheumatic fever. Unlike the fever of Still's disease the temperature remains raised throughout the day. The presence of fever or its recurrence is a good indicator of the activity of rheumatic fever.

Arthritis. Arthritis and fever are the commonest clinical features and are usually the presenting symptoms. Arthritis occurs in the large joints although the small joints of the hands and feet can be affected. Typically it is described as a flitting or migratory arthritis. In the affected joint there is pain, tenderness and swelling, which usually lasts for only a few days but as it subsides in one joint similar symptoms and signs develop elsewhere. It is rare for more than a few joints to be involved at the same time. X-rays show no erosive changes and there is no permanent damage to the joints. This migratory polyarthritis may continue for some weeks and exceptionally for some months.

```
          Arthritis

      1. Flitting
      2. Large joints
```

Carditis. This is the most important feature of rheumatic fever because of the possiblity of permanent damage to the valves of the heart. All three layers of the heart, the endocardium, myocardium and pericardium, may be affected. Heart involvement occurs in about 50% of cases of rheumatic fever and of those who have heart involvement 50% will have some degree of permanent damage to the heart valve. Tachycardia is common in rheumatic fever and may simply reflect the fever but a sleeping pulse rate of over 100 suggests that there may be some myocardial involvement. Involvement of the pericardium produces pericarditis with chest pain and an audible pericardial rub on ausculation. Later there may be pericardial effusion which will be demonstrated on X-ray of the chest by a rapid increase in the size of the heart. It is rare for the effusion to be large enough to need draining. All valves of the heart may be affected but the most frequently affected are the mitral valve followed by the aortic valve. Involvement of the valves is demonstrated by the emergence of murmurs on ausculation. The ECG may also be abnormal. In the most severe cases congestive heart failure may follow but death from this cause is rare in the first attack of rheumatic fever but is the usual cause of death in recurrent attacks. In adults many cases of mitral and aortic valve disease give no history of rheumatic fever in childhood but it is thought that the damaged valves are a consequence of a childhood attack of rheumatic fever which was so mild as to be undiagnosed at that time.

Carditis

1. Pericardial effusion
2. Damage to valves, mainly mitral and aortic
3. Myocarditis

Chorea. Chorea may occur alone without any of the other manifestations of rheumatic fever. It is a self-limiting condition and leaves no permanent disability. Chorea consists of sudden, uncoordinated and involuntary movements. These may affect the face, tongue, limbs and trunk. In its mildest form it is easy to overlook, the child merely appearing to be rather clumsy but in severe forms there may be extremely violent movements which the child is totally unable to control. Most of the involuntary movements stop during sleep. Attacks last from a few days to a few months and may recur.

The skin. The skin is affected in about 10% of patients with rheumatic fever by erythema marginatum, also called erythema annulare and erythema circinatum. The skin shows a pink rash with a pale centre and an irregular outline which gradually spreads outwards. The rings are usually seen on the trunk and may vary from a single to multiple lesions. They do not itch and usually fade within a few days but may recur later in the illness.

Nodules. These are usually a later complication of rheumatic fever and are rare if the heart is not involved. They are hard, mobile, non-tender, sub-cutaneous masses, usually appearing over the scalp, elbows, knees and ankles. They differ from the nodules of rheumatoid arthritis in that they are smaller and tend to occur in groups. They also differ on microscopic appearance in that they show none of the palisading of cells seen in the rheumatoid nodule.

Laboratory investigations

There is no specific laboratory test for rheumatic fever. The ESR is almost invariably raised although this is in no way diagnostic. However, it may be useful in following the disease activity, a falling ESR being associated with decreasing activity of the rheumatic fever.

The antistreptolysin titre (ASOT) will be raised in about 80% of children with rheumatic fever but it should be noted that a negative result when first tested does not exclude the diagnosis, for it may be some weeks before the values become abnormal. A raised ASO titre is not diagnostic of rheumatic fever, only of a recent streptococcal infection. The SCAT and Latex tests are always negative. There may be a mild to moderate degree of anaemia.

Differential diagnosis

Still's disease. There may at times be considerable difficulty in diagnosis in the early stages of both diseases. In Still's disease there is more often involvement of the peripheral joints of the hands and feet and the resultant swelling is more persistent than the flitting arthritis of rheumatic fever. In Still's disease the temperature is usually remittent, ie it returns to normal at some time during each day. In both conditions there may be a skin rash but in Still's disease the lesions are smaller than in rheumatic fever and do not expand outwards. Chorea is never associated with Still's disease and valvular damage to the heart does not occur in Still's disease. In the older child the SCAT test may be positive in juvenile rheumatoid arthritis.

Osteomyelitis. Osteomyelitis, particularly if it occurs near to a joint, may be associated with pain in that joint and an effusion. However, it is rare for more than one joint to be affected and maximum tenderness may be demonstrated a short distance away from the joint. In the early stages the X-ray will be normal and the ESR will be raised. If there is any doubt blood cultures may need to be carried out.

Henoch-Schoenlein purpura. This may be associated with joint pain and swelling and the characteristic petechial rash may not appear for some time but when it does it establishes the diagnosis.

'Growing pains'. Pains in the limbs, usually the legs, and often worse at night, are quite common in children and are called by the parents 'growing pains'. The exact nature of these pains is uncertain but there is no systemic illness, ie no fever, nothing abnormal is found on clinical examination and the BSR is normal.

Viral infections. The common viral infections in childhood, such as chicken-pox and measles, are frequently associated with arthralgia and less commonly with arthritis but the previous history of skin rash and the transient nature of the joint symptoms should not cause confusions.

Differential Diagnosis of Rheumatic Fever

1. Still's disease and rheumatoid arthritis
2. Osteomyelitis
3. Henoch-Schoenlein purpura
4. 'Growing pains'
5. Arthralgia of fevers

Treatment:

This can be divided into two sections, treatment of the episode of rheumatic fever and treatment aimed at preventing further attacks.

Treatment of the acute attack consists of bed rest, aspirin or steroids and penicillin. The exact importance of bed rest is uncertain. Traditionally this consisted of total rest in bed for many months; nowadays there is a tendency to reduce the period of bed rest and to allow the child to move around within the bed without restraint. Most people agree that bed rest should be continued as long as there is any evidence of active carditis or a raised temperature. The child may then be allowed up for short periods each day and his response to the increased activity noted and if there is any evidence of deterioration, bed rest may need to be resumed. In this way the child is gradually mobilized but after discharge from hospital will probably need to spend some weeks at home before returning to school. Whether any physical restriction should be placed on a child who has had carditis or who has a persistent pathological murmur is debatable.

Aspirin is given to control the fever. There is no evidence that it influences the outcome of the disease in any way. It is given in sufficient dosage to produce a blood level of around 25 mg/100 ml. Steroids are no more effective than aspirin in the long term but are more effective in suppressing the signs of disease activity and may therefore be indicated in the presence of active carditis. Both drugs are continued until there is no clinical evidence of disease activity when they can be slowly withdrawn and the child observed closely to see that there is no flare-up of the disease activity. Although rheumatic fever is due to previous, rather than concurrent, infection with haemolytic streptococci, it is customary to give a ten day course of antibiotics (usually penicillin) to make sure that all the organisms have been killed.

Prevention of further attacks is very important and all patients should take a prophylactic antibiotic (usually an oral penicillin) for at least five years after the attack or until they leave school, whichever is the longer.

Treatment of Rheumatic Fever

1. Bed rest
2. Aspirin
3. Steroids
4. Antibiotics
      Acute attack
      Prophylactically for at least 5 years

Henoch–Schoenlein Purpura (anaphylactoid purpura)

This is a disease of unknown aetiology associated with non-thrombocytopenic purpura.

Aetiology

This is unknown, although some cases seem to follow haemolytic streptococcal infection, while others seem to have an 'allergic' basis to drugs or insect bites.

Clinical features

Hencoh–Schoenlein purpura occurs in children, usually before the age of six. The onset is acute and joint symptoms or skin rash or abdominal pain may be the presenting symptom. The rash is usually most striking over the buttocks and consists of red macules with petechiae; similar changes are commonly seen on the back of the legs. The rash fades in seven to ten days without leaving any scar. The knee joints are commonly involved and sometimes also the ankles, other joints are rarely affected. The joints are painful and swollen for only a few days.

Abdominal pain is usually colicky and this is thought to be due to a haematoma developing in the bowel wall. Occasionally an intussusception of the bowel occurs.

Laboratory investigations

There are no specific changes. The most important negative results are a normal platelet count with normal bleeding and clotting times. The ESR is raised and sometimes also the ASO titre. The SCAT and Latex tests are negative.

Complications

About 10% of patients develop an acute nephritis with haematuria and albuminuria and this may become chronic.

Treatment

Only symptomatic treatment is required for those cases that do not develop a nephritis but the urine needs to be checked daily and if proteinuria or haematuria develop, steroids should be started. Death, which is uncommon, is due either to nephritis or intussusception. Occasional patients are seen in whom there are several recurrences but most patients recover, having had only one attack.

Henoch-Schoenlein Purpura

1. A non-thrombocytopenic purpura with skin rash and petechiae
2. Abdominal colic from haematoma of bowel wall
3. Mild joint pain and swelling
4. Only important complication – acute nephritis

Erythema Nodosum

Erythema nodosum is a skin lesion which may be associated with several other diseases or may occur by itself without obvious cause.

Aetiology

Erythema nodosum used to be associated most often with primary tuberculous infection but as this has become less common, it is now more often associated with sarcoidosis, streptococcal infection, ulcerative colitis, Crohn's disease or certain drugs. The skin lesions are not due to the direct presence of any bacteria but probably represent an allergic type of response.

Clinical features

Erythema nodosum usually occurs in children and young adults. The typical skin lesion is red, raised above the skin, firm and tender. These nearly always occur over the front of the legs but occasionally similar lesions are seen on the arms. Over a few days the lesions change colour to a yellow-blue bruised appearance and then gradually fade away. There may be only a single lesion or several lesions may occur together or succeed each other over several weeks. About one-third of cases are associated with an arthralgia and in some of these there is a transient synovitis, commonly of the knees and ankles. There is no permanent joint damage. Joint symptoms usually settle in a few days but sometimes persist for a few weeks.

Laboratory investigations

A search has to be made for any primary cause. A chest X-ray and a Mantoux test should be carried out. The ASO titre will be raised if there has been a preceding streptococcal infection. The ESR is usually raised but the SCAT and Latex tests are negative.

Treatment

In the absence of any primary cause, treatment is with aspirin for any joint symptoms. Occasionally, when there is recurrent erythema nodosum over several months, steroids may be used.

Erythema Nodosum

1. Due to:
   Primary TB
   Sarcoid
   Streptococcal infection
   Drugs
   Idiopathic
2. Skin lesion: usually on legs
3. Self-limiting

8
Other Inflammatory
Types of Arthritis

Systemic Lupus Erythematosus

Systemic lupus erythematosus (SLE) is currently thought to be an auto-immune disease which may affect many organs in the body (multisystem disease) and is associated with the presence of 'anti-nuclear antibodies'.

Aetiology

In auto-immune disease the body behaves as though it is allergic to its own tissues and becomes self destructive. Damage may occur to the joints, muscles, nerves' skin, kidneys, lungs, etc. Associated with this damage, many different types of antibodies may be demonstrated in the patient's blood, anti-nuclear factor (ANF), anti-DNA and antilymphocyte antibodies being common.

After taking certain drugs, particularly hydrallazine (which is used for the treatment of hypertension), procainamide, some anti-tuberculous drugs and certain sulphonamides, some patients develop an illness that resembles systemic lupus in that there may be fever, arthralgia or arthritis with pericarditis and pleural effusions. Occasionally LE cells are found. This illness, however, differs from true SLE because (1) it clears up on withdrawal of the drug, (2) renal involvement does not occur, and (3) anti-DNA antibodies are not found.

Discoid lupus is a chronic skin condition associated with an erythematous scaly rash, usually on the face, which heals by scarring. It is now becoming apparent that some of these cases also have mild systemic involvement and occasionally have a positive LE cell test, and this disease probably represents the mildest form of the spectrum of systemic lupus.

Pathology

Almost any organ in the body can be affected. In order of descending frequency these can be ranged as joints, skin, kidney, lymph glands, heart, lungs, liver, spleen and brain. Joint symptoms occur in approximately 90% of patients and skin lesions in about 80%, whereas brain damage occurs in only about 20%. Blood vessels may become the site of vasculitis producing similar clinical effects to those seen in rheumatoid arthritis. SLE is approximately nine times more common in women than in men. The onset may be at any age from childhood onwards, but most cases occur between the ages of twenty and forty. Occasional cases have a history of sensitivity to sunlight with a tendency for the disease to flare up after undue exposure to the sun.

Clinical Features

With the possibility of such widespread organ involvement, many different clinical patterns of SLE can occur. Joint symptoms being very common, many cases first present to the rheumatologist with a history of arthralgia or of arthritis. In many ways the arthritis resembles rheumatoid arthritis in that it is usually peripheral and symmetrical (ie involves the hands and feet). However, it differs from rheumatoid arthritis in that erosions are relatively uncommon so that serious bone damage to the joint is rare. Nevertheless, contractures around the joint do occur, producing both swan neck and Boutonnière deformities identical to those seen in rheumatoid arthritis. Early in the disease, when there is no skin involvement and the patient presents with arthritis alone, it may be impossible to differentiate from rheumatoid arthritis. In both conditions the sheep cell agglutination and ANF tests may be positive and LE cells may not be seen early in the disease. Suspicion that systemic lupus is the cause of joint symptoms may be aroused by a history of a previous illness involving the heart, lungs or kidneys or by finding leucopenia on laboratory testing. Further confusion can arise as nodules may occur in both conditions, although they are very rare in systemic lupus and common in rheumatoid arthritis.

The classical skin rash is described as having a butterfly distribution, spreading across both cheeks and the bridge of the nose (Fig. 8.1). Although not always present it is virtually diagnostic. A great variety of other skin rashes with erythema, papules and purpura may occur but are much less specific for diagnostic purposes.

Renal involvement is demonstrated by the presence of proteinuria, which if sufficiently severe can lead to a nephrotic syndrome and later renal failure. Microscopy of the urine may show red cells and casts.

The heart may be affected by pericarditis. Occasionally the valves of the heart are affected, a condition known as Libman–Sacks endocarditis, and heart murmurs may develop, although these never produce serious mechanical problems.

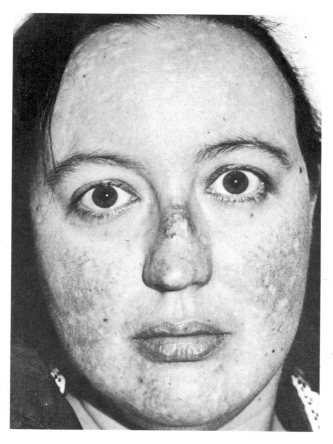

Fig. 8.1 Butterfly rash of systemic lupus erythematosus.

Pleurisy occurs in approximately 50% of cases of lupus and the lungs are sometimes involved in a pneumonitis, which shows on X-ray as patchy areas similar in appearance to bronchopneumonia but not responding to antibiotics.

Psychiatric complication may indicate underlying disease of the brain. Depression, anxiety or more gross psychotic illness may be present. Organic brain disease may present with epilepsy, hemiplegia or other neurological signs. Death from neurological involvement is becoming increasingly important.

Systemic Lupus Erythematosus

1. Men to women ratio 1:9
2. Any age: maximum incidence 20–40 years of age
3. Multi-organ disease
   Skin/butterfly rash
   Joints
   Kidneys
   Brain
4. Presence of anti-nuclear antibodies
5. Demonstration of LE cells

Laboratory Findings

Some degree of anaemia is common. This is usually non-specific but occasionally antibodies to red blood cells cause a haemolytic anaemia and then the Coombe's test will be positive. The white blood cells often show some depression with a total white blood count falling perhaps to 2000/ml. The ESR is usually raised and the SCAT may be positive. The ANF test is usually positive throughout the course of the disease and LE cells will be seen usually at some time during the illness but are not constant. Serum complement levels may be reduced and anti-DNA antibodies raised in active disease. If there is renal involvement a renal biopsy may provide confirmation of the diagnosis and give some guidance as to the prognosis of the renal disease.

Differential Diagnosis

Obviously with a potential involvement of so many different organs in the body the differential diagnosis may cover the whole of medicine. The rheumatologist is mainly concerned with the differential diagnosis of lupus from other forms of arthritis (see Table 8.1). The presence of a butterfly rash is diagnostic but LE cells are seen in other types of arthritis and other diseases. Just as syphilis is regarded as the great mimic in general medicine, SLE may be regarded as the great mimic in arthritis and may enter into the differential diagnosis of most forms of inflammatory joint disease.

Table 8.1 Differential Diagnosis between Rheumatoid Arthritis and SLE

	Rheumatoid Arthritis	*Lupus*
Nodules	Common	Rare
Erosions	Common	Rare
LE cells present	10%	80%
ANF test positive	20%	100%
Complement level	Normal	Decreased
Anti-DNA antibodies	Normal	Increased with nephritis

Natural History

The severity of the disease may vary from a mild illness with transient arthralgia to a most severe disease with rapid involvement of many organs and death occurring within a few years. In the past SLE had a very poor prognosis, many patients dying within a few years of the diagnosis being made. However, with modern methods of treatment many of the features of SLE may be controlled. In addition, the newer and more sensitive tests for anti-nuclear antibodies are allowing the diagnosis to be made in many milder cases whose prognosis is good. Nowadays the common causes of death are renal failure, CNS involvement or overwhelming infection.

Treatment

Patients with SLE may react in an allergic manner to almost any drug. Drugs should therefore not be given without careful consideration as to their likely benefit. In the milder forms with arthritis as the major disease manifestation, perhaps associated with skin rash, chloroquine phosphate is often very effective. In addition, aspirin can be given to control joint pains and stiffness. Gold should not be used, as it may make the disease worse. Local treatment to affected joints is similar to that of rheumatoid arthritis with rest of the joints, splintage, hydro-cortisone injections, exercises, etc.

Any evidence of involvement of organs other than the joints is usually an indication to start steroid therapy and this may need to be given in high doses (80 mg prednisolone per day at times). In these cases azathioprine is sometimes used in addition in an attempt to reduce the steroid dosage. With high dosage of steroids infection is a constant hazard and needs to be borne in mind if the patient develops any fresh symptoms.

Pregnancy is not contra-indicated in SLE although, unlike

rheumatoid arthritis, joint symptoms do not usually improve during pregnancy and occasionally the disease may flare up, particularly if there is renal damage.

Polymyalgia Rheumatica and Giant Cell Arteritis

This is a disease of unknown aetiology, occurring in the elderly and presenting with pain and stiffness in the joints around the shoulders and hips. In some cases there is an associated giant cell arteritis.

Pathology

Although the patient complains of intense pain and stiffness in the muscles, the muscles are normal. Microscopy shows no abnormality, the muscle enzymes in the blood are normal and the electromyelogram is also normal. It is possible that the symptoms are coming from inflammation of the small joints around the shoulder and the small joints of the spine in the cervical and lumbar areas.

Clinical Features

The main features are pain and severe stiffness around the shoulders and hips. Pain is usually bilateral but occasionally starts unilaterally and is worse with movement but there is often a continuous dull ache. Early morning stiffness at these sites may be very severe. Frequently patients say that they are unable to get out of bed unaided in the morning because of this stiffness. The stiffness usually passes off after several hours, but in severe cases may last until mid-afternoon only to return in the evening after sitting. The onset in some cases is so acute that the patient can name the day of onset; more usually the illness develops over a few days and less commonly over a few weeks. On examination at this stage there is little abnormal to find, except for some limitation of movement at the shoulders and hips caused by pain. In the more severe forms of polymyalgia, there is a systemic illness with fever, loss of appetite, loss of weight and malaise. Within a few weeks patients may appear to have a terminal illness because of these marked systemic disturbances.

Giant Cell Arteritis

Giant cell arteritis may affect any medium or large size artery in the body; because it frequently affects the temporal artery it was at one time known as temporal arteritis. There is inflammation throughout the wall of the artery and occasional very large cells with many nucleii are seen (giant cells). The vessel may be occluded causing infarction of the tissues supplied by the artery. Symptoms from the arteritis depend upon which vessels are affected. The temporal arteries cause headache with pain over the affected vessel. Blindness is not uncommon due to arteritis of the retinal artery. Other complications may be cerebral thrombosis, myocardial infarction and necrosis of bowel. If the temporal vessels are involved there is often visible enlargement and tenderness. Arteritis at most other sites has to be inferred from the patient's symptoms as the vessels cannot be examined.

Giant cell arteritis may occur by itself but about 40% of patients with polymyalgia rheumatica have, in addition, giant cell arteritis.

Polymyalgia Rheumatica

1. Occurs in the elderly
2. Pain and stiffness around shoulders and hips
3. May be systemic illness
4. 40% have giant cell arteritis

Laboratory Investigations

There is no specific laboratory test for the diagnosis of polymyalgia rheumatica. An almost constant feature is a raised ESR, often over 100 mm/hr. There may be a non-specific anaemia; the SCAT is negative and LE cells are not seen. X-rays show no erosive changes but changes of cervical and lumbar spondylosis are common because of the age of the patient and serve only to confuse the diagnosis.

Differential Diagnosis

A large number of diseases may be considered in the differential diagnosis.

1. Rheumatoid arthritis usually starts in the peripheral joints and is associated with erosive changes on X-ray and a positive SCAT. Nodules never occur in polymyalgia rheumatica.

2. Osteoarthrosis. Some degree of osteoarthrosis is common in the elderly but OA is never associated with severe early morning stiffness or a raised ESR.

3. Polymyositis and dermatomyositis cause weakness of muscles rather than stiffness and are associated with raised muscle enzymes in the blood (SGOT, SGPT, CPK, Aldolase).

4. Psychogenic. Because of the lack of physical signs it may be felt that there is no organic disease present but a raised ESR excludes a psychogenic cause.

5. Carcinomatosis and myeloma may cause skeletal pains and be associated with weight loss and malaise. X-rays will eventually show changes although these may take time to develop. Marked early morning stiffness is not a feature of either condition.

Treatment

Mild cases of polymyalgia without evidence of arteritis may be treated with analgesics such as aspirin or indomethacin (Indocid) but a close watch needs to be kept on the patient to diagnose arteritis if it develops. Polymyalgia associated with systemic features or arteritis should be treated with steroids in a sufficient dose to reduce the ESR to below 20 mm/hr. Initially this may need quite high doses of prednisolone but this can be reduced if the ESR falls. Polymyalgia is a self-limiting disease and usually remits spontaneously after 18 months to 5 years. At intervals, therefore, the steroid dosage can be reduced and the ESR checked; any rise means a return to the previous dosage of prednisolone. Using this technique most patients should eventually be weaned off steroids.

Polyarteritis Nodosa (PN)

This is an inflammatory condition affecting medium sized arteries and smaller arterioles, the lesions are segmental in distribution with normal areas of vessel in between; any artery in the body may be affected.

Aetiology

This is unknown, although occasional cases have followed the taking of penicillin and sulphonamides. It has been suggested that this is another example of an auto-immune disease.

Pathology

Polyarteritis nodosa is more common in men than women, in a ration of 4:1. It may occur at any age but is commonest in young adults. In the affected artery there is inflammation extending throughout the arterial wall and the artery may be occluded either by thrombosis at this site or from thickening of the vessel wall. Healing is by fibrosis with scarring of the vessel wall and further constriction of the lumen may occur at this stage. The veins are also sometimes affected, when the term vasculitis should be used instead of arteritis. The outlook is poor; most cases despite treatment die within five years of the diagnosis although occasional cases can go into a complete spontaneous remission.

Clinical Features

Systemic features with a fever, malaise, loss of appetite and loss of weight may occur. Like SLE other features depend upon the organs which are involved.

Skin. It may be possible to palpate the nodules in the arteries underlying the skin. In addition there may be infarction of the fingers or toes and leg ulcers may develop. Various types of non-specific skin rash may also occur.

Lungs. The lungs are involved in about 30% of patients and may be the first site to be affected. Early symptoms are coughing and shortness of breath and a diagnosis of bronchitis or asthma may be made at this stage. With more advanced disease there may be multiple areas of lung infarction with secondary infection and the formation of lung abscesses with cavities visible on X-ray.

Kidney. This is probably the most commonly affected organ and early signs are proteinuria and microscopic haematuria. Hypertension is usual with long-standing polyarteritis nodosa and a common cause of death is renal failure.

Cardio-vascular system. Apart from hypertension, myocardial infarction may occur from involvement of the coronary vessels.

Gastro-intestinal system. Vague abdominal pain is common. Infarction may occur in the bowel, liver and pancreas.

Central nervous system. As in SLE there may be a wide range of symptoms and signs. Hemiplegia, epilepsy, disturbances of sensation and involvement of peripheral nerves with sudden paralysis of isolated peripheral nerves (known as mononeuritis multiplex) may occur. Sudden blindness may be due to involvement of the retinal artery.

Joints. Arthralgia is common, true synovitis is much more rare.

Muscles. Muscle pain with tenderness and weakness is quite common and is due to involvement of the arterioles within the muscles.

Laboratory Investigations

The ESR is almost always raised in the active stage of the disease. In contrast to SLE the white blood count is usually raised and occasionally there is a very marked eosinophilia. SCAT and Latex tests are nearly always negative. A biopsy of an affected artery is really essential for the diagnosis and this is preferably from an organ that is known to be involved, such as the skin or kidney. If this is not possible a 'blind' muscle biopsy may show the typical changes within the arteriole.

```
            Polyarteritis Nodosa

        1. Men to women ratio 4:1
        2. Maximum incidence in young adults
        3. Patchy inflammation of arteries
           and occasionally also veins
        4. Multi-organ disease
              Lungs
              Kidneys
              CNS
              Muscles
```

Differential Diagnosis

Like SLE a large number of medical conditions may be considered in the diagnosis. The multi-system involvement associated with a high ESR may first suggest the diagnosis.

Treatment

Treatment is usually with steroids but they are not as fully effective as in SLE. High doses may be required but the dosage should gradually be reduced if the disease comes under control. Hypertension may need treating. Immuno-suppressive drugs such as azathioprine are sometimes used in addition to steroids in the most severe cases.

Polymyositis and Dermatomyositis*

Polymyositis is an inflammatory condition of unknown aetiology affecting muscles; if associated with changes in the skin the condition is called dermatomyositis.

Pathology

Both polymyositis and dermatomyositis may occur at any age and the sexes are about equally affected. In adults, but not in children, there is an increased frequency of malignant growths associated with both conditions; malignant growths have variously been reported as occurring in 20–70% of cases. These may not be found when the myositis is first diagnosed and their removal is not always associated with an improvement in the muscle disease. The exact relationship between malignancy and myositis remains to be discovered. Early in the disease the muscles may be swollen from the inflammation but later become wasted and contracted. Calcification may occur in the muscles, skin and sub-cutaneous tissues. Joint involvement is rare.

Some cases develop the skin changes seen in scleroderma and in others there is a picture of a 'mixed connective tissue disease' (MCTD) with some of the features of myositis, scleroderma, LE cells and Sjögren's syndrome, all appearing in the same patient.

The prognosis for myositis and dermatomyositis in children is probably better than in adults. In adults the prognosis seems worse for the elderly patient, who more often has an associated neoplasm.

Polymyositis and Dermatomyositis

1. Occur at any age
2. In adults associated with an increased incidence of carcinoma
3. Symptoms are muscle weakness and tenderness

---

*Myopathy, myositis and dystrophy. Dystrophy is applied to those disorders of muscles which are inherited, ie pseudo-hypertrophic muscular dystrophy. Myositis is applied where there is evidence of inflammation in the muscles, ie dermatomyositis. Myopathy may be used to cover all types of muscle disease and in this case dermatomyositis could be called an inflammatory type of myopathy. However, some authors restrict its uses to non-inflammatory, non-inherited muscle disease, ie thyrotoxic myopathy.

Clinical Features

The onset is usually insidious and the major symptoms are weakness and tenderness of muscles. This usually starts around the shoulders and hips. The patient may notice difficulty in getting up from a squatting position or difficulty in holding objects above the head. The neck muscles are frequently affected but the facial muscles are usually not involved. As the disease spreads the muscles of respiration may be affected and also those involved in speech and swallowing. Early in the disease there is little muscle wasting but the muscles may be tender and rather firm or woody when palpated. Later muscle wasting becomes marked and as contractures of the muscles develop joint deformities occur. Arthralgia is usually present but synovitis in the joints is rare.

The classical skin change associated with dermatomyositis is a lilac discoloration of the upper eyelids. Changes elsewhere in the skin are less specific but there may be thickening and erythema and sometimes a scaly rash is seen over the knuckles and fingers. Calcification may occur and may be palpable in the skin or sub-cutaneous tissues. Areas of calcification may break down and leave a discharging sinus.

Death is usually due to respiratory paralysis or malnutrition and infection.

Laboratory Results

The ESR is often raised but a normal ESR does not exclude the diagnosis. Serum globulin level is usually raised and occasionally the SCAT is positive. Muscle enzyme levels (SGOT, SGPT, CPK and Aldolase) are raised in the presence of active disease and falling values indicate a response to treatment.

X-rays may show calcification in the skin; erosions in the joints are rare. Electromyographic studies (EMG) may be helpful in making the diagnosis and often skin and muscle biopsies are taken for the same reason.

Treatment

Steroids are usually prescribed in an attempt to reduce the severity of the disease, although they often have to be given in high doses and improvement does not always follow. If improvement occurs the dosage of prednisolone can be reduced slowly to that level which just controls the patient's symptoms and this can be checked by serial studies of the muscle enzymes. Azathioprine, cyclophosphamide or methotrexate may be added to the treatment in the hope that it will allow a reduction in the dose of prednisolone.

Polymyositis and Dermatomyositis	
Laboratory	1. Raised muscle enzymes
	2. Typical biopsy appearance of affected muscles
	3. EMG
Treatment	Steroids
Prognosis	Poor, particularly if carcinoma is present

Physiotherapy is aimed at avoiding or minimizing contractures by splintage of joints. Exercises may help improve the power of non-affected muscles. The occupational therapist may be able to help the patient with more severe deformities.

Systemic Sclerosis

Systemic sclerosis is a chronic disease characterized by a hard, firm thickening of the skin and associated with changes in other organs particularly bowel and kidney. In the past this condition was known as scleroderma but with the recognition of the widespread involvement of other organs it is more appropriately known nowadays as systemic sclerosis.

Pathology

Systemic sclerosis is more than twice as common in women as in men. Although it may occur at any age, including childhood, it usually develops between twenty and fifty. The relationship of systemic sclerosis to dermatomyositis is uncertain; certainly cases of dermatomyositis are seen which then go on to develop all the features of systemic sclerosis. Apart from the skin, there may be involvement of the lungs, kidneys and gastro-intestinal tract. In the latter there is a loss of mobility from sclerosis of the bowel walls, so that the gut becomes an atonic tube, leading to constipation and malabsorption. Although synovitis may occur in the joints, severe damage does not occur and erosions are rare.

Clinical Features

One of the earliest symptoms is the development of Raynaud's phenomena. Raynaud's phenomena can occur without being associated with any other disease but in these cases there is often a family history and symptoms start in the teens. Adult onset Raynaud's phenomena is often associated with a variety of rheumatic diseases. In Raynaud's phenomena there is a spasm of the arterioles of the fingers on exposure to cold and the fingers go through a colour sequence of white to blue to red when warmed.

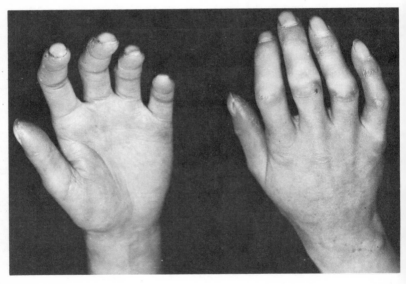

Fig. 8.2 Hands in systemic sclerosis. Note tightness of skin over fingers and scars at the tips of the fingers.

Other early symptoms are a polyarthritis affecting the hands and non-pitting oedema of the skin over the fingers. Later the skin becomes sclerotic and movements in the underlying joints are lost through tightness of the skin (Fig. 8.2). Eventually a claw-like, rigid hand develops and permanent reduction of the blood supply associated with the sclerosis produces ischaemia of the hands, leading frequently to gangrene of individual fingers. Similar changes develop in the feet.

An unusual feature that may suggest the diagnosis is a palpable and sometimes audible creaking over the tendons and joints as they move.

Skin changes may develop over the trunk and face as well as over the limbs. On the face the mouth becomes puckered and cannot be fully opened and the nose becomes thin and prominent. Facial expression is lost through the skin changes and the face assumes a characteristic mask-like appearance at all times. Calcification commonly appears in the skin and telangiectasia are common when sclerosis has developed.

The commonest gastro-intestinal symptom is dyspepsia from oesophagitis associated with reflux of gastric acid into the oesophagus. Involvement of the lower bowel may lead to malabsorption and constipation which may be extreme and life threatening.

About 30% of patients show diffuse fibrosis on X-ray of the chest. Symptoms are usually less severe than the X-ray suggests.

Severe and at times malignant hypertension may develop. Renal failure may occur and kidney involvement is a common cause of death.

The muscles may be involved with a myositis, although this can be difficult to detect, because of the overlying changes in the skin.

Systemic Sclerosis

1. Occurs mainly in young women
2. Skin—sclerosis, loss of joint movement, gangrene of fingertips
3. Lungs—fibrosis
4. Bowels—loss of peristalsis with malabsorption
5. Kidneys—hypertension and renal failure

Laboratory Investigations

The ESR is usually raised, as is the serum globulin. The LE cell test is occasionally positive and the SCAT more often positive. The ANF test may be positive in up to 50% of cases. There is no specific laboratory test diagnostic of this condition other than biopsy of an involved area of skin.

X-rays of the hands and feet may show, in those cases with marked

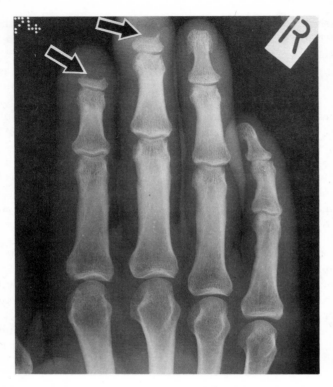

Fig. 8.3 X-ray of hands in systemic sclerosis. Note absorption of terminal phalanges (arrowed).

ischaemia, a typical appearance with absorption of the distal phalanges (Fig. 8.3). A barium swallow may show loss of peristalsis of the oesophagus and this may be seen in the absence of symptoms.

Treatment

There is no known treatment for this condition. Steroids used early in the disease may reduce the initial arthritis in the hands and feet but do not influence the progression of the skin changes. Ischaemic lesions of the hands and feet may be reduced by wearing warm gloves and stockings when exposed to cold. Hypertension may need treatment if it is severe. Attempts should be made to improve the malabsorption.

Although occasional cases may remit, most cases have a poor prognosis with death occurring within 10 years of the initial diagnosis. Occasional cases are seen which have been slowly progressive over twenty years.

Systemic Sclerosis

1. No effective treatment known
2. Prognosis poor

9
Infective Forms of Arthritis

Infections of joints may occur with bacteria, viruses and occasionally fungi.

Bacterial Infection

Bacterial infection is usually secondary to infection elsewhere but can occur from direct penetrating injury to the joint. Common sites of primary infection are the skin (boils and other septic conditions),

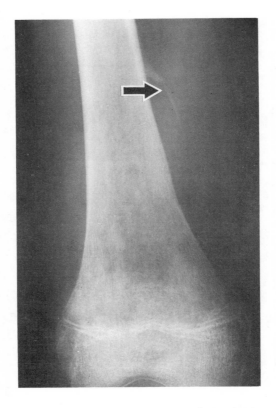

Fig. 9.1 Osteomyelitis. The arrow points to the periostium which has been lifted off the bone by underlying pus. In this case the joint was not infected.

teeth with root abscesses and the urinary tract. Sometimes the joint is infected from an area of osteomyelitis, situated within the joint capsule. The following types of bacterial infections will be considered:

(1) Pyogenic arthritis
(2) Gonorrhoea
(3) Tuberculous arthritis
(4) Brucellosis

Pyogenic arthritis

Many organisms have been isolated from infected joints but the common ones are staphylococci, streptococci, *H. influenzae, E. coli* and proteus. In adults it is common to find that the affected joint is the site of pre-existing inflammatory polyarthritis (commonly RA); in children the joint usually has no pre-existing disease. Treatment of inflammarory polyarthritis with steroids is associated with an increased incidence of pyogenic infection of the joints. Untreated infection leads to severe damage to the cartilage and bones in the involved joint. Symptoms are usually acute with fever and often rigors. Usually only one joint is affected (commonly the knee) and shows warmth, redness of the overlying skin, tenderness and extreme pain on attempted movement. This typical picture of an inflammatory process may be much reduced in the rheumatoid patient; the signs may be much less dramatic and it is a useful rule to aspirate any joint which suddenly 'flares up' in rheumatoid disease to exclude infection. Patients being treated with steroids may show only a minimal response to bacterial infection. The presence of rigors indicates that septicaemia is occurring.

Pyogenic Arthritis

1. Usually secondary to infection elsewhere
2. Usually staphylococcal infection
3. Acute onset, sometimes with rigors
4. Severe joint pain
5. All symptoms and signs greatly reduced if patient is taking steroids

---

The essential investigation is aspiration and culture of synovial fluid from the affected joint. Routinely, blood cultures should be done in addition. The ESR will be elevated as is the white cell count. X-rays are normal in the early stages of pyogenic arthritis and nowadays most cases are diagnosed before X-ray changes are visible.

If the joint is extremely painful it is more comfortable in a full plaster cylinder, which should have a window cut out to allow access to the joint for further aspiration. Once aspiration and blood cultures have been taken broad spectrum antibiotics can be started and changed if need be when the results of culture and sensitivity testing are known. Most antibiotics pass freely into the synovial fluid so that intra-articular injections are not essential; but if the joint is being aspirated it is reasonable to inject antibiotics at the end of the procedure. Antibiotics need to be continued for at least six weeks after the symptoms have settled to prevent recurrence. As the infection of the joint settles, the splint can be removed and passive joint movements should be started. Pyogenic arthritis, treated early, has a good prognosis but if diagnosed late, some permanent damage to the joint will occur and some loss of movement is common.

Gonococcal arthritis

Gonococcal arthritis is secondary to gonococcal infection elsewhere, usually the genito-urinary tract. Joint involvement is uncommon if cases of gonorrhoea are treated early. In the joints there is a pyogenic arthritis which may affect several joints or be mono-articular, in which case the knee is often the affected joint. Symptoms develop two or three weeks after the initial infection. There is usually a systemic illness with fever and malaise. The affected joint is swollen, warm and tender. A specific skin lesion may be found, a small (3–5 mm) red papule which contains the gonococcus and represents a septic skin infarct. There may be only one lesion or several may be found.

Diagnosis depends on isolating the gonococcus from the synovial fluid and, in addition, cultures of blood and any urethral discharge should be carried out. The gonococcal complement fixation test, if positive, only indicates that the patient has had gonorrhoea at some time in the past and if negative does not exclude current gonococcal infection.

Gonococcal Arthritis

1. Secondary to gonococcal infection elsewhere
2. Usually only one or two joints involved
3. Systemic illness
4. Skin lesions

Treatment is similar to that described for pyogenic arthritis and most cases are sensitive to penicillin. With prompt diagnosis the prognosis for the affected joint is good. A venereologist should be involved in the management of these cases as he has special facilities for tracing contacts and thus reducing the spread of gonorrhoea.

Tuberculous arthritis

Tuberculous infection of bones and joints is secondary to infection elsewhere, usually either in the lungs or genito-urinary tract. It used to be commonest in young children but is now seen at all ages and may affect joints also affected by other forms of inflammatory arthritis. As in pyogenic arthritis, steroids may increase the risk of tuberculous arthritis developing.

Three common sites of infection are hips, knees and spine. Spinal tuberculosis (Pott's disease) usually develops in the dorsal area; the lesion starts in one vertebra and may spread upwards and downwards and a cold abscess may develop and track out along muscle sheaths to the surface.

In the hips and knees, joint involvement may be secondary to nearby osteomyelitis. There is marked proliferation of the synovium which erodes underlying cartilage and bone. Effusions tend to be small. Eventually the infection extends through the joint capsule and may form a sinus to the skin. If not treated promptly and adequately fibrous or bony ankylosis develops.

Clinically there may be features of a systemic illness with pyrexia, malaise, loss of appetite, loss of weight and in particular night sweats. Symptoms from spinal lesions may be vague until there is bony collapse and instability of the spine and possibly neurological damage due to cord compression. In the peripheral joints there is pain, swelling and reduced movement. There may be a tuberculous tenosynovitis of tendons around the joint.

Tuberculous Arthritis

1. Secondary to infection elsewhere
2. Destruction of vertebrae and discs in spine
3. In peripheral joints X-rays show marked osteoporosis and later bone destruction
4. Sinuses may develop
5. Treatment with anti-tuberculous drugs plus surgery

The essential diagnostic test is to demonstrate the presence in the spine or peripheral joints of tubercle bacilli. This usually means an open biopsy. The Mantoux test, if positive, only means a primary infection has occurred but, if negative, does to some extent weigh against a diagnostic of tuberculous infection. X-rays early in the disease show only osteoporosis of the bones. Later the peripheral joints show loss of space with erosions. Spinal lesions may show an abscess within the vertebrae and later collapse of one or more vertebrae.

Treatment is usually a combination of anti-tuberculous drug therapy with surgery. In the peripheral joints surgery is aimed at removing excess synovium and any necrotic bone. In the spine, removal of necrotic bone may be followed by surgical fusion of the affected vertebrae. Management of spinal tuberculosis may mean a long period of bed rest on a plaster body shell. Drug treatment needs to be continued for many months.

Brucellosis

Three strains of brucella, present in animals, may cause an infection in man. *Brucella melitensis* occurs in goats, *B. abortus* occurs in cows and *B. suis* occurs in pigs. In Great Britain, *B. abortus* occurs through drinking untreated cows' milk. Vets who treat aborting cows may also become affected. There is a systemic illness with fever, malaise, loss of appetite and loss of weight, which develops about three weeks after drinking the infected milk. Infection of bones and joints may occur and causes destructive lesions in bones and joints similar in many ways to tuberculous infection. Diagnosis may be difficult to establish as the organisms are not easily isolated from infected sites. Agglutination tests on the patient's serum may show a rise in antibodies to brucella.

Treatment is by prolonged courses of antibiotics and if there is extensive bone damage, surgical exploration and drainage.

Viral infections

The common viral infections of childhood, rubella, mumps, influenza and upper respiratory tract infections are often associated with arthralgia and occasionally with a mild transient synovitis in some joint. No permanent damage occurs. The importance of these symptoms and signs lies in the fact that they may cause some confusion with Still's disease or rheumatic fever. However, the short duration of symptoms and signs reveals their benign nature.

Viral hepatitis and glandular fever are sometimes associated with arthralgia and more rarely arthritis. The arthritis is self limiting and causes no permanent damage to the joint or joints.

Fungal infections

Fungal infections may be secondary and occur during prolonged antibiotic treatment of septic arthritis or osteomyelitis. Primary infections are uncommon and usually involve several organs in the body besides the bones and joints. X-rays may show extensive destructive changes which may cause confusion with osteomyelitis or tuberculosis. The diagnosis depends on culturing the fungus from the infected site.

Further Reading

Outline of Orthopaedics 4th rev. edn., by J. Crawford Adams (Churchill Livingstone).

10
Soft Tissue Rheumatism

This term encompasses a number of common painful conditions which arise in soft tissue often around a joint. Like osteoarthrosis they are predominantly diseases of middle and old age.

Soft Tissue Rheumatism

Shoulder syndromes
    Rotator cuff lesions
    Frozen shoulder
    Bicipital tendonitis

Elbow epicondylitis
    Tennis and golfer's elbow

Plantar fasciitis

Fibrositis

Sudek's atrophy (reflex sympathetic dystrophy)

Bursitis and tenosynovitis

Dupuytren's contracture

Periarthritis of the shoulder and anatomy of the shoulder joint

This term includes a number of painful conditions which arise from soft tissue lesions around the shoulder joint. To understand these conditions more fully, some basic anatomy is necessary (Fig. 10.1).

The shoulder is a ball and socket joint with the ball being the head of the humerus and the socket the shallow glenoid of the scapula. The humerus is held in position mainly by muscles. The rotator cuff is a group of muscles arising from the scapula and inserted around the neck of the humerus into the capsule and tuberosities. These muscles form a cuff around the shoulder joint. The muscle most frequently involved in periarthritis is the supraspinatus muscle which arises from just above the scapula spine and passes beneath the acromium to be inserted into the capsule and greater tuberosity of the humerus. This muscle is separated from the acromium and the deltoid muscle by the subacromial bursa. The action of the muscle is to initiate abduction, ie moving the arm out from the side of the body. The rest of abduction is carried out by the large deltoid muscle which arises

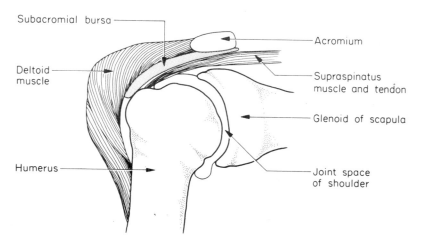

Subacromial bursa

Deltoid muscle

Humerus

Acromium

Supraspinatus muscle and tendon

Glenoid of scapula

Joint space of shoulder

Fig. 10.1 Diagram of shoulder joint and related structures.

from the acromium, overlies the supraspinatus muscle and bursa and is inserted into the humerus lower down.

Rotator cuff lesions

Degeneration of the supraspinatous tendon is common in the older age groups. This makes the tendon more liable to tear with minor trauma which may, in fact, pass unnoticed and the onset of pain may appear spontaneous. Pain is felt mainly at the point of the shoulder with radiation down the arm. It may be very severe and often causes insomnia. The usual course is that over a matter of weeks or months the condition gradually subsides. A few go on to develop a more generalized stiff shoulder. The physical sign is pain on abducting the arm causing the classical painful arc of movement. Pain is caused by the tender tendon rubbing against the acromium. Simple movements such as putting on a coat or hanging things up become very painful and difficult. Treatment is by subacromial injection of corticosteroid and local anaesthetic and when the pain has settled by gentle exercises to mobilize the shoulder and prevent stiffness.

Direct trauma or sudden exertion may completely rupture the supraspinatous tendon. The patient then suffers a sudden shoulder pain and finds abduction of the shoulder very difficult. The tear may heal and in the elderly it is treated conservatively. In young people, however, in which this is an unusual injury, the tear should be repaired surgically.

In a small number of cases supraspinatus lesions are associated with the laying down of calcium salts in the tendon. This is called acute calcific tendonitis.

Frozen shoulder (adhesive capsulitis)

This is a condition in which shoulder pain is associated with painful and restricted movement of the gleno-humeral joint in all directions. In severe cases the joint may become completely immobile, ie frozen. The natural history of the condition is for the pain and stiffness to subside gradually over a matter of months, although complete movement may not be regained. Frequently the condition is bilateral although the onset is seldom synchronous. In many cases the condition arises spontaneously. In others, however, it is secondary to trauma, a stroke or myocardial infarction. Treatment is often ineffectual although analgesics are necessary to relieve pain. Attempts to maintain shoulder movements with physiotherapy are worthwhile and applications of ice or heat have analgesic properties. Sometimes improvement is obtained by manipulation under anaesthetic.

Bicipital tendonitis

This is an unusual cause of painful shoulder due to inflammation of the long head of the biceps as it passes across the humeral head. Local steroid injections are the most appropriate treatment.

Elbow epicondylitis (tennis and golfer's elbow)

These conditions comprise pain and tenderness over the epicondyles of the elbow. The lateral epicondyle is the most frequently affected and has the label 'tennis elbow'. The peak age of onset is between forty and fifty and perhaps represents a clash between continuing high levels of physical activity and the onset of musculo-skeletal degeneration. The pain appears to arise from the origin of the extensor muscles of the forearm. In the case of golfer's elbow, it is the origin of the flexor muscles on the medial epicondyle which is painful. The condition may arise spontaneously or follow exertion, eg playing tennis or closing heavy van doors or it may follow a direct knock on the elbow. If spontaneous it may be isolated or may be part of a more generalized fibrositic syndrome or associated with cervical spondylosis. A few cases of tennis elbow are thought to be due to entrapment of the posterior interosseous nerve.

The pain may be severe with radiation both up and down the arm and occasionally paraesthesiae in the fingers. Gripping is much affected and pain may occur at night.

Treatment is by resting the arm in a sling and in the case of tennis elbow a cock-up splint may help; by local infiltration of corticosteroids; by physical methods such as ultrasound and friction. Sometimes surgery is needed to release the extensor origin. Although treatment is initially usually successful, recurrence does occur in at least a third of cases.

Plantar fasciitis

Painful heels occur in broadly two groups of people. Firstly, patients with ankylosing spondylitis or other sero-negative arthritides may develop tender, painful heels which are associated with eroded calcaneal spurs on X-ray. The second and commoner group are people usually middle-aged and overweight who do a lot of walking on pavements, eg postmen. These people develop tender heels without eroded calcaneal spurs. Treatment is by wearing heel pads and local steroid injections into the tender area. In the case of a sero-negative arthritis, anti-inflammatory drugs like phenylbutazone or indomethacin may help. The condition tends to improve gradually over one to two years.

Fibrositis

This is a chronic painful condition presenting as pain and tenderness along the trapezius muscles and in the paraspinal areas of the lower cervical and mid dorsal spines. Painful trigger spots at the elbow epicondyles, around the shoulders and around the sacro-iliac joints are common. The cause of fibrositis is unknown. It is so called because at one time it was believed to be due to inflammation of small nodules in soft tissues particularly the trapezius muscles. Important factors in the aetiology of fibrositis are believed to be cervical and dorsal spondylosis and the tendency to develop a chronic tension state with ensuing muscle spasm and insomnia. Treatment is symptomatic and consists of local heat, injections of trigger spots with local anaesthetic and steroid, analgesia and adequate night-time sedation to correct the insomnia. Techniques of relaxation are worth trying. Counselling is essential to establish whether there is a remedial cause of stress in the patient's life.

Sudek's atrophy (shoulder-hand syndrome, disuse atrophy, reflex sympathetic dystrophy)

This is a condition characterized by pain, diffuse swelling and vaso-motor changes occurring in a limb. The number of names that this condition has, testifies to the obscurity of the exact cause and pathogenesis. Despite the localizing name of shoulder-hand syndrome, Sudek's atrophy may also involve the foot and leg. It is commonly post-traumatic though it may be associated with other conditions.

Causes of Sudek's Atrophy

1. Spontaneous
2. Post-traumatic
3. Cervical spondylosis
4. Myocardial infarction
5. Hemiplegia
6. Associated with consumption of certain drugs, eg anticonvulsants

---

The usual sequence of events is that following an injury the limb becomes stiff and painful to move. The pain seems out of proportion to the injury and there may be cutaneous hyperalgesia. Diffuse swelling of the affected part occurs. The skin appears smooth, mottled and cyanotic and feels cold. Inappropriate sweating occurs. Even when the condition follows a definite injury to the involved limb, similar but less marked changes may be detected in the uninjured contralateral limb. A characteristic osteoporotic mottling of bone occurs on X-ray. The disease may go on to severe muscle and bone wasting with contractures of soft tissues. The majority recover over one to two years. Treatment is aimed at preventing immobilization and maintaining as much activity as possible. In the hand this is best achieved by task-orientated mobilization in an occupational therapy workshop. Similar activity with the legs, eg on pedal machines, can be supplemented with hydrotherapy. Passive exercises and correction of contractures with plasters are of help. A wide variety of drugs have been used and advocated. Oral corticosteroids are said to produce remission. Blocking sympathetic pathways by stellate ganglion block also has its advocates. However, one has a strong impression that at best, treatment prevents further deterioration whilst natural recovery occurs.

Bursitis and tenosynovitis

Inflammation of synovial tissue found outside joints is usually included under soft tissue rheumatism.

Bursitis

A bursa is a sac of synovial tissue which develops over or between the pressure of moving parts. Sometimes these bursa become inflamed due to trauma, especially occupational trauma. They may also be involved in systemic arthritides and swell and become inflamed in gout and rheumatoid arthritis. Common sites of bursitis are as follows:

(1) Subacromial bursitis.
(2) Olecranon bursitis. The bursa at the elbow is frequently involved in rheumatoid arthritis or gout.
(3) Pre-patellar bursitis. The bursa in front of the patella becomes swollen and painful in certain occupations involving excessive kneeling, eg 'housemaid's knee' and the 'beat' knees of coalminers.
(4) Ischial bursitis. Inflammation of the ischial bursa used to be common in weavers and was known as weaver's bottom and was apparently due to prolonged sitting on hard surfaces. It occasionally presents as a spontaneous onset of bursitis.
(5) Bursa between the tendo-Achilles and the hindfoot is another site of pain.

Treatment of bursitis consists of removing the cause wherever possible and secondly, local steroid injections into the inflamed bursae. Other physical methods of treatment may be tried and in some cases surgical excision of the bursa is necessary.

Tenosynovitis

Synovial tubes in which tendons run may become inflamed in rheumatoid arthritis but sometimes in otherwise healthy people. In this group the cause is usually some awkward repetitive movement. A common site for tenosynovitis is at the wrist and involves the long extensor and abductor tendons of the thumb. Tenderness, pain and swelling is experienced on the radial side of the wrist associated with movement of the thumb. This condition is known as De Quervain's tenosynovitis. Treatment is by local steroid injections into the tendon sheaths and immobilization for three weeks in a splint or by surgical release.

In the hand, the flexor tendons run in fibrous tunnels on the palmar surface of the fingers. The mouths of these tunnels may become constricted and a swelling forms on the tendon. This causes obstruction to the free play of tendon through the tunnel and extending the finger is accompanied by a click as the nodule clicks through the narrow mouth of the tunnel. The condition is known as trigger finger or stenosing tenosynovitis. A similar phenomenon occurs in rheumatoid arthritis, where the synovial lining of the tendons becomes involved in the rheumatoid process. Again treatment is by local injections of corticosteroid into the tendon sheath and if this is ineffective then surgical opening of the mouth of the tendon tunnel is required.

Dupuytren's contracture

In this condition there is a thickening and contraction of the deep soft tissues in the palm of the hand. This results in an increasing fixed flexion of the fingers beginning with the little finger.

Treatment is by operation. Dupuytren's contracture may be associated with pads on the knuckles (Garrod's knuckle pads). It may be familial and there is an association with alcoholism.

Carpal Tunnel Syndrome (C.T.S.)

Compression of the median nerve as it passes through the carpal tunnel at the wrist results in the carpal tunnel syndrome. This comprises tingling and numbness in the thumb and first two fingers, characteristically worse at night and on waking. If no treatment is given muscle weakness may eventually occur in the hand.

The carpal tunnel syndrome occurs in pregnancy and may be the presenting feature of hypothyroidism or arthritis of the wrist. Often no obvious cause can be found.

Treatment is by local corticosteroid injection into the carpal tunnel or by splinting the wrist at night or by surgical decompression.

Further reading

'Diagnosis of Soft Tissue Lesions', by J. Cyriax, In *Textbook of Orthopaedic Medicine*, vol. 1. (Baillière Tindall)
'Non-articular rheumatism and the fibrositis syndrome', by H. A. Smythe, In *Arthritis and Allied Conditions*, eds. J. L. Hollander and D. J. McCarthy. (Lea and Febiger)

11
Bone Disease

Symptoms of bone disease may be mistaken for arthritis, and diseases of mineral metabolism and bone may in turn cause inflammatory arthritis and secondary osteoarthritis.

It is important to realize that the skeleton although performing an essential supporting and mechanical role also has the equally important function of being a reservoir of calcium and other minerals which are essential for the correct function of tissues such as nerve and muscle. In the metabolic bone diseases these roles may clash and the skeleton may become starved of minerals in order to maintain correct levels of calcium. It is also important to realize that bone is not a static tissue but is constantly being destroyed (resorption) and formed.

This chapter is not a comprehensive survey of bone disease but reflects those diseases that are likely to be seen in rheumatological practice.

Hyperparathyroidism

The essential abnormality in hyperparathyroidism is the overproduction of parathyroid hormone. This hormone is produced by the four parathyroid glands in the neck; its function is to maintain a normal blood calcium. A stimulus to production of the hormone is a lowering of the blood calcium. Parathyroid hormone increases blood calcium mainly by removing calcium from the bones and also by its action on the kidney and by its effect on vitamin D metabolism. The hormone may be produced in excess from tumours of the glands (adenoma and carcinoma), and by enlargement of all the glands (hyperplasia). This is known as primary hyperparathyroidism. Secondary hyperparathyroidism is overproduction of the hormone

Hyperparathyroidism	
Primary:	due to parathyroid tumours or hyperplasia
Secondary:	due to chronic renal failure, osteomalacia

due to the stimulus of a low blood calcium (hypocalcaemia). The most common cause of this is vitamin D deficiency, and vitamin D resistance which occurs in chronic renal failure.

A sustained increase of parathyroid hormone for whatever reason will result in a loss of mineral from bone, causing bone weakness. In primary hyperparathyroidism the high levels of blood calcium will also result in calcification in the kidney, and in the production of renal stones. The clinical results of primary hyperparathyroidism are epitomized under the eponym of bones, stones and groans. The loss of mineral from the bone may result in cysts and fibrosis of the bone (osteitis fibrosa cystica). This causes diffuse pain in the limb and chronic gnawing pains in the back. The bones are tender. Fractures (Fig. 11.1) and deformities occur and teeth may fall out.

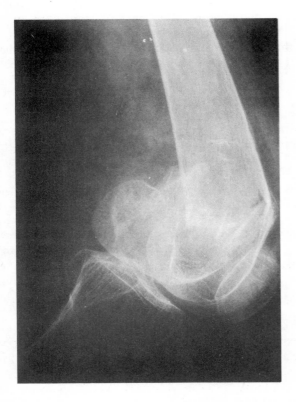

Fig. 11.1 Pathological fracture of the femur above the knee in a woman with hyperparathyroidism.

Hypercalcaemia itself produces symptoms such as loss of appetite, nausea, vomiting and constipation. Muscle weakness occurs and the patient passes large amounts of urine. Mental changes occur and patients have been diagnosed only after admission to psychiatric units.

Stones form in the renal tract and the patient may present with renal colic. Renal failure occurs due to obstruction by the stones or due to the calcification of kidney tissue. Calcification may also occur in joint cartilage (chondrocalcinosis), and results in attacks of pseudogout.

Results of Primary Hyperparathyroidism

Hypercalcaemia
Renal calcification and stone formation
Osteitis fibrosa cystica
Chondrocalcinosis and pseudogout

Diagnosis

Diagnosis is made by considering the possibility of the disease when confronted with a patient with any of the above symptoms and specifically by measuring the blood calcium and phosphate. In a case of primary hyperparathyroidism the serum calcium is raised and the serum phosphate is low. In secondary hyperparathyroidism serum calcium will be within the normal range and the serum phosphate will depend on the cause of the secondary hyperparathyroidism. If due to lack of vitamin D, the phosphate will be low but in chronic renal failure it will be raised. X-rays of the hands show a characteristic picture of excessive bone resorption.

Treatment

Treatment of the primary form is removal of the tumour or hyperplastic glands. Post-operatively the patient may suffer from tetany due to a sudden fall in blood calcium, and calcium supplements and high doses of vitamin D are necessary. Secondary forms are treated by treating the cause where possible.

Osteomalacia

Bone is composed of an organic matrix made up of collagen fibres and mucopolysaccharides. This gristly substance is made hard by the deposition of calcium salts on the collagen fibres. This is the process of ossification and the resulting hard firm structure is what we call bone. Failure of this process is called rickets in children and osteomalacia in adults. Vitamin D is necessary for the process of calcification and in most cases of rickets and osteomalacia it is lack or relative lack of vitamin D which is at fault.

Vitamin D is found in the diet particularly in eggs, margarine, dairy produce, liver and fish oils. It is also made in the skin by the action of ultraviolet light on a cholesterol derivative. Before it is active the vitamin has to be processed by the liver and then the kidneys. The active principal has the name of 1:25 dihydroxy-cholecalciferol (125 OHC). This substance is essential for the absorption of calcium by the gut and for the calcification of osteoid as explained above. The requirements for an adult vary in relation to the amount of sunlight exposure. The more one is exposed to sunlight the less vitamin D one needs to take in one's diet. The requirement for an adult can be estimated as being from 100 to 500 MRC units a day. It follows, therefore, that osteomalacia may be caused by a lack of sunlight, by not eating the right foods, by malnutrition or by an inability to absorb vitamin D even if the right foods are eaten. Liver and particularly renal disease may interfere with the processing of vitamin D despite adequate amounts being absorbed.

Causes of rickets and osteomalacia

1. *Lack of vitamin D*
   Lack of sunlight
   Lack of vitamin D in the diet
   Gut disease with the inability to absorb
   vitamin D
2. *Vitamin D resistance*
   Chronic renal failure
   Congenital renal tubular abnormalities,
   eg Fanconi's syndrome and renal tubular
   acidosis

In particular osteomalacia and rickets may be caused by an absolute lack of vitamin D in a poor diet, because of food fads or poverty, and by lack of sunlight reaching the skin. Often the two reasons co-exist especially in the elderly recluse. It may also be caused by an excessive need for vitamin D in pregnancy and lactation where large amounts of calcium are passed to the fetus and baby. It is rare in the affluent countries of the west but common if repeated pregnancies take place with a poor diet.

Gut diseases which interfere with absorption of vitamin D also result in osteomalacia. Examples of these are coeliac disease, Crohn's disease and obstructive jaundice where bile acids do not reach the intestinal contents. Osteomalacia is not uncommon in patients who have undergone gastrectomy.

In chronic renal failure the damaged kidneys are incapable of converting the vitamin D absorbed or made in the skin into the active principal 1:25 OHC. In the congenital diseases of renal tubular function the main abnormality is an excessive loss of mineral, especially phosphate, via the kidneys despite the otherwise normal functioning of vitamin D metabolism. In renal tubular acidosis the renal tubules are incapable of getting rid of excess acid and this interferes with the calcification of osteoid.

Clinical Features

Rickets. In children lack of vitamin D results in a series of bony deformities. Enlargement and tenderness of bone ends simulate arthropathy (Fig. 11.2). Bossing of the skull and abnormalities of the ribs with classical bowing of the legs due to bending of the soft tibia and femur, occur. The disease is now rare in patients of European stock, but is seen in children of Asian immigrants. In babies and very young children rickets may present as tetany and convulsions.

Osteomalacia. In adults the common presenting symptoms is bone pain felt particularly in the back and the legs. Pain is worse on weight bearing and moving. The bones may be exquisitely tender. Sudden pain may be due to a fracture which can occur spontaneously or with minimal trauma. Muscle weakness due to lack of vitamin D may be severely incapacitating (vitamin D deficient myopathy). In severe osteomalacia with a very low blood calcium, tetany may occur. This is spontaneous twitching of muscles and may be associated with mental changes. Radiographs show thin bones and characteristic lesions known as Looser's zones or pseudo-fractures. These are seen

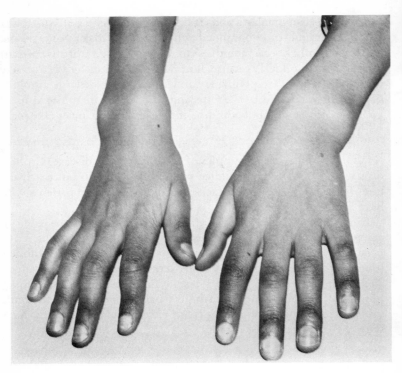

Fig. 11.2 Rickets. The wrists appear swollen due to enlargement of the lower end of the ulna and radius.

particularly along the lateral edges of the scapula, in the rami of the pubic bones and in the necks of the femurs. Blood tests show a normal or low calcium concentration and low or normal serum phosphate and an elevated alkaline phosphatase.

Treatment

Treatment is by correcting the deficiency of vitamin D. This is easily done by vitamin D supplements in the deficiency types of osteomalacia and rickets. However, in vitamin D resistance such as occurs in chronic renal failures, very high doses of vitamin D may be necessary or alternatively, in patients with chronic renal failure new synthetic forms of 125 OHC can be used (1 alpha OHC). In some of the renal tubular defects complicated regimens to correct mineral and acid base abnormalities are necessary. The danger of vitamin D treatment is that it may produce hypercalcaemia and when patients are on vitamin D, symptoms of hypercalcaemia should be watched for and the blood levels of calcium checked periodically.

Renal osteodystrophy

This is a term used to describe the bone disease associated with chronic renal failure. Essentially it is a combination of osteomalacia as described above and secondary hyperparathyroidism.

Osteoporosis

This is a state where there is a lack of bone substance but the bone present is normal. This distinguishes it from the previously described diseases where the lack of bone is associated with changes in bone structure.

Lack of bone with age is so common that it is often difficult to say whether we are dealing with a disease or a natural ageing process. We all lose bone from the third decade onwards due to the fact that bone is being resorbed faster than it is being laid down. Osteoporosis, however, may be called a disease when the amount of bone present is inadequate for the needs of the body so that normal physical activities result in a spontaneous fracture.

Causes of Osteoporosis

1. Menopause
2. Disuse
3. Endocrine: Corticosteroid excess due to Cushing's disease or to administration of steroids
Thyrotoxicosis
4. Gastrectomy

1. Post-menopausal. The rate of bone loss in women tends to accelerate over the menopause. If the menopause is artificial and sudden, ie caused by removing or irradiating the ovaries this effect is exaggerated. It would seem that the female sex hormones produced by the ovaries exert a protective effect on bone and the loss of them leads to excessive resorption. However, it must be stressed that this is by no means universal and many women do not suffer from osteoporosis after either a normal or surgical menopause.

2. Disuse. Osteoporosis is an inevitable consequence of disuse. This applies to a limb, part of a limb or the whole body. Resting in a splint or disuse because of a painful joint will both result in osteoporosis. Stroke and paraplegia by producing paralysis have similar effects on the affected limbs. One of the disadvantages of bed rest is the risk of generalized osteoporosis. Disuse osteoporosis is however reversible if activity is regained in the affected part and to some extent it can be corrected even during rest if muscle action is combined with non-weight bearing. Disuse osteoporosis is an important contribution towards the osteoporosis that one often finds in patients with rheumatoid arthritis of long duration.

3. Endocrine. The most important endocrine cause of osteoporosis is Cushing's syndrome. This syndrome is caused by excessive secretion of cortisol by the adrenals. It is a relatively rare disease but its effects are seen unhappily and more frequently when corticosteroids are given as therapy, eg in rheumatoid arthritis, asthma and other conditions. The effect is dose related but not inevitable, eg if a small dose of steroids enables a patient to move around more then the beneficial effect of increased activity on the bone will outweigh the osteoporotic effect of the drug. The effect may also be lessened by giving the steroids on alternate days.

Clinical features

The clinical effects of osteoporosis are fractures and loss of height. The noticeable sites of fracture are the wrist, femoral neck and vertebrae. In the vertebrae the fractures are described as crush fractures (Fig. 11.3) and these occur particularly in the dorsal spine whereas in the lumbar spine the intervertebral discs are seen to balloon into the fragile vertebrae. The fractures are seen in elderly women rather than men largely because of the accelerated loss of bone over the post-menopausal years. Fractures may result from trivial injuries. Healing occurs normally and treatment is on conventional orthopaedic principles. Crush fractures of the vertebrae are treated by bed rest, prone lying, and analgesics until the major pain has settled. The effect of repeated vertebral fractures is a gradual loss of spinal height. Over the years this results in permanent skin creases forming round the waist and a dorsal kyphosis (Duchess' hump) and eventually the rib cage may overlap the pelvis.

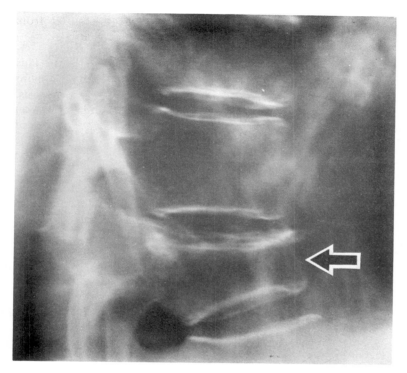

Fig. 11.3 Osteoporosis. The arrowed vertebra has undergone a crush fracture due to osteoporosis. Compare height of vertebra with one above.

Treatment

The treatment of osteoporosis is controversial and a number of different methods have been tried.

1. Female sex hormones. These have been shown to decrease bone loss after oophorectomy if given within three years of the operation. It is therefore reasonable to treat post-menopausal osteoporosis with hormone replacement treatment (HRT) especially if indicated on other grounds, eg flushing. Oestrogens do carry a risk of thromboembolic disease.

2. Fluoride. Sodium fluoride increases the amount of bone in the skeleton and indeed if consumed in excess results in a disease known as fluorosis where bones become brittle and very dense on X-ray. However, when given with vitamin D and calcium it has been claimed that good new bone is laid down and vertebral fractures decrease.

3. Other drugs, such as anabolic steroids, calcium and calcitonin have been used in the past and are probably ineffectual.

4. In the elderly with osteoporosis, osteomalacia may also be present and a supplement of vitamin D such as calcium and vitamin D tablets is worthwhile.

5. Prevention is better than cure and a practical way of preventing osteoporosis is to encourage activity even in people who are crippled with arthritis.

Paget's disease of bone

This condition is caused by excessive bone resorption which is equalled by excessive new bone formation. This overactive bone metabolism may operate at twenty times the normal rate. The effect of this overactivity is to produce bone laid down in a disorderly manner. The effect on individual bones is that they become softer,

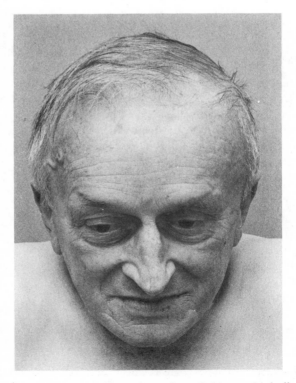

Fig. 11.4 Paget's disease of bone has enlarged this man's skull.

deformed, more liable to fracture and very vascular. One or many bones (polyostotic) may become involved. The disease commonly involves the skull (Fig. 11.4), vertebrae, pelvis, femurs and tibiae. It is predominantly a disease of the elderly and the prevalence increases with age. It may run in families. Commonly there are no symptoms and the condition is discovered accidentally in one or more bones on X-ray.

Complications in Paget's disease

1. Bone pain
2. Arthrosis
3. Fractures
4. Nerve compression
5. Heart failure
6. Malignant change
7. Renal stones on bed rest

Complications

Sometimes pain seems to arise in the bone itself because of the softening or increased metabolic activity. Alteration of joint structure such as in the hip causes a form of secondary osteoarthrosis. The abnormal bones may break spontaneously or with a minimal trauma, and transverse fractures across long bones occur. The deformed enlarged bones may press on nerves in the skull causing blindness and deafness and in the spine causing spinal cord and nerve compression resulting in tetra- and paraplegias. The greatly increased blood flowing through these bones can cause a form of congestive heart failure when a large proportion of the skeleton is involved. In a very small proportion of people the disease may become malignant with the formation of a bone sarcoma. This is usually accompanied by the onset of, or a great increase in, pain. Diagnosis of Paget's disease is confirmed by the characteristic X-ray picture and by a raised serum alkaline phosphatase.

Treatment

There have been many attempts to interfere with the overactive bone metabolism including the use of steroids, aspirin, anti-cancer drugs, radiation and fluoride. The current remedy is to give injections of calcitonin.

Calcitonin is a hormone produced naturally by the C cells of the thyroid gland. Its action is to some extent the opposite of parathyroid hormone in that it decreases the resorption of bone and decreases the concentration of serum calcium. The compound used therapeutically may be derived from salmon, pigs, or may be a synthesized human type. The dose is expressed in MRC units and a common dose for Paget's disease would be 50 to 100 MRC units a day intramuscularly. In Paget's disease a course of calcitonin injections may be expected to decrease the bone metabolism with a concomitant decrease in bone pain and a fall in serum alkaline phosphatase. It is necessary to continue the injections indefinitely. There have been claims that both nerve compression and heart failure as well as bone pain respond to this treatment. Arthritis of the hip may be treated by the usual analgesics, physical measures and joint replacement. Fractures are treated along normal orthopaedic lines and heal well.

Inherited disorders of bone

There are many such diseases most of which are very rare. A few are described below.

Osteogenesis imperfecta. This is an inherited disorder of bone in which the bones are brittle and liable to fracture. The condition may present at birth, in childhood or in later years when it appears as premature osteoporosis. It may be associated with blueness of the whites of the eyes and sometimes deafness supervenes in the late teens. The severity varies greatly from patient to patient, some children being severely stunted and crippled by multiple and frequent fractures, whilst others merely fracture their bones rather more easily than their peers. The cause is an abnormality of collagen. There is no definite medical treatment but much is required and can be achieved in the way of social, educational and medical rehabilitation.

Achondroplasia. In this inherited condition there is a failure of ossification of cartilage. The result is a normal sized skull, small face, short limbs and normal trunk. These people often earn their living as circus dwarfs. There is a tendency for them to develop spinal stenosis.

Mucopolysaccharidoses (Hurler's, Hunter's, Sanfilipo's and Scheie's syndromes). These are a set of rare inherited abnormalities of connective tissue in which excess amounts of mucopolysaccharide are produced. The results vary from one syndrome to another but include mental retardation, eye and other CNS complications, gross bone deformity and cardiac abnormalities. Scheie's syndrome may be confused with Still's disease.

Bone malignancies

Tumours in bone may cause bone pain and present in a rheumatic clinic. The most common tumours are metastases secondary to carcinomas elsewhere, especially from the breast, prostate, kidney and thyroid gland.

Myelomatosis. This is another malignancy which may present with bone pain. It is predominantly a disease of the elderly and is due to the malignant overgrowth of plasma cells in the bone marrow. These cells produce an abnormal protein which can be diagnosed on serum electrophoresis (see Chapter 13, p. 157) or reveals itself as Bence Jones proteinuria.

12
Miscellaneous Conditions

Aseptic necrosis

Aseptic necrosis (avascular necrosis) of bone is thought to be due to infarction of a segment of bone. Usually this affects the femoral head but may involve other sites, particularly the tibial condyles of the knee joint. It may occur without obvious cause in a normal joint but more often the joint is the site of an inflammatory arthritis (RA and SLE). It has been suggested that it is more common after treatment with steroids. Rarer causes are decompression sickness in divers, sickle cell disease of the blood and alcoholism.

```
Causes of Aseptic Necrosis

1. Rheumatoid arthritis
2. SLE
3. Steroid drugs
4. Decompression sickness
5. Sickle cell disease
6. Excessive alcohol intake
```

The onset is usually acute with pain and limitation of movement in the joint. X-rays are normal at first but later show condensation of an area of bone and later still, collapse of the bone in this area. Rapid destruction of the joint may occur. There is no specific treatment but in the hips and knees weight bearing should be avoided during the acutely painful stage. If there is extensive destruction then arthroplasty may be needed later.

Chondromalacia patellae

This term is used to describe a group of symptoms which are not uncommon. It may be that there are several different pathologies accounting for the symptoms. Although it is thought that the symptoms arise from the patella, at times on inspection at surgery no abnormality can be seen.

The patient is usually a young adult and more commonly female. The symptoms, pain in the knee and occasional swelling, are usually worse after exercise or prolonged periods of standing. On examination there may be a small effusion and rocking the patella on the underlying femoral condyles may be painful, as also may be palpation of the under-surface of the patella. X-rays are usually normal.

Treatment is ill-defined. That activity which precipitates symptoms should, if possible, be avoided. Injections of hydro-cortisone into the joint seem on occasions to help. With severe and persistent symptoms patellectomy has been undertaken but without controlled trials remains unproven in effectiveness.

Hypertrophic osteoarthropathy

This is characterized by clubbing of the fingers (Fig. 12.1), arthritis of the peripheral joints and periostitis of the affected bones. Rare congenital cases do occur but the disease is usually associated with

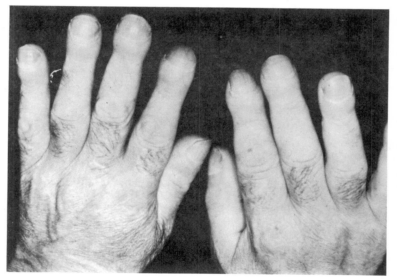

Fig. 12.1 Clubbing of fingers in hypertrophic osteoarthropathy.

carcinoma of the lung or pleura (Fig. 12.2). Other causes are chronic chest infection, cirrhosis of the liver and malabsorption. In addition to the clubbing of the finger tips, there is usually a complaint of arthralgia and sometimes there is a synovitis in the affected joint. The essential diagnostic feature is the presence on X-ray of periostitis (Fig. 12.3), particularly over the radius and ulna at the wrist.

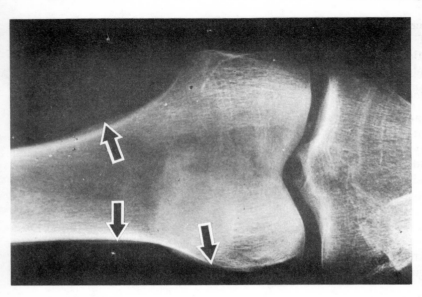

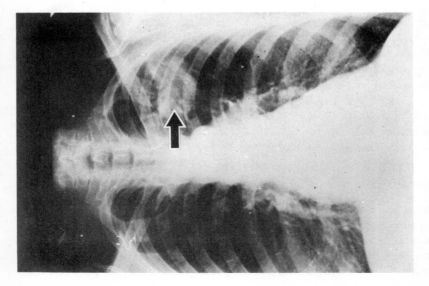

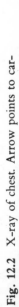

Fig. 12.3 X-ray showing periostitis around knee

Fig. 12.2 X-ray of chest. Arrow points to car-

Removal of the tumour or radiation is often associated with relief of joint symptoms. If operation is impossible analgesic/anti-inflammatory drugs or steroids may give symptomatic relief.

Blood diseases associated with joint symptoms

Haemophilia and Christmas disease. These are inherited disorders with defective clotting of the blood. Bleeding may occur into any joint after very mild trauma. Blood is an irritant within the joint and sets up an inflammatory response. The onset is acute with pain and swelling of the affected joint. Repeated attacks in the same joint can lead to fibrous ankylosis and severe degenerative changes. In the acute stage the appropriate clotting deficiency factor in the blood should be replaced. Local treatment to the joint consists of rest, possibly with splintage, and then gradual mobilization as symptoms settle to prevent deformity. There is doubt whether aspiration of the joint does more harm than good.

Sickle cell disease. This is an inherited disease confined to negroes and characterized by an abnormal type of haemoglobin in the blood. This causes the cells to assume a 'sickle shape' in the presence of a low oxygen concentration in the blood. Sickle cells tend to clump together and cause obstruction in the blood vessels, leading to infarction of the tissues. Joint symptoms are common and may be due to infarction of bone (avascular necrosis). This commonly affects the hands and feet, although any joint may be affected.

Thalassaemia. This is another inherited disorder with an abnormal type of haemoglobin but there are no specific joint symptoms unless there is an element of sickle cell disease associated with it.

Leukaemia. Particularly in children, acute leukaemia can cause bone pain, arthralgia and sometimes synovitis. There may be confusion with Still's disease.

Sarcoidosis

Acute sarcoidosis may present with erythema nodosum and frequently there is an arthralgia and sometimes a true synovitis is present as well. Chest X-ray usually shows bilateral enlargement of the hilar lymph glands. This type of sarcoid is usually self-limiting and settles within two years. Occasional cases become chronic and some are chronic from the start and give no history of erythema nodosum. In these cases there may be a peripheral and symmetrical arthritis, similar to rheumatoid arthritis or isolated large joint involvement. Biopsy of the synovium shows a typical appearance of sarcoid granuloma. X-rays show cystic lesions around the joint margins. Treatment is usually with steroids.

Neuropathic joints (Charcot's joints)

In diabetes mellitus, tabes dorsalis and syringomyelia, there is reduced or absent pain sensation from the joints. This is associated with a picture of extreme damage to the joints. On X-ray there are gross destructive changes with massive osteophytes. Clinically there is usually a marked deformity of the joint, with bony enlargement and considerable crepitus on movement. The changes are often most marked in the knees.

Palindromic rheumatism

This presents with a history of recurrent attacks of acute arthritis, usually involving only one joint in each attack. Between attacks the ESR is normal, the SCAT is negative and X-rays show no bony damage. Some of these cases eventually develop into established rheumatoid arthritis or SLE. However, some continue to have repeated attacks without permanent joint damage over many years.

Individual attacks are treated along standard lines with anti-inflammatory drugs. Chloroquine phosphate is sometimes effective in reducing the frequency of the attacks.

Intermittent hydrarthrosis

This presents as recurring effusions, usually in the knees. The usual age of onset is between 15 and 45 years. Attacks tend to recur at a fairly constant rate. No permanent joint damage occurs.

13
The Laboratory in Rheumatology

The laboratory plays an important role in the diagnosis and monitoring of patients with rheumatic diseases. Various laboratory tests with special relevance to such patients will be described.

Haematology

Haemoglobin concentration (Hb). Normal: men 13.0 to 17.0 g/100 ml, women 12.0 to 15.5 g/100 ml. Anaemia can be defined as a low concentration of haemoglobin in the blood. Anaemia is common in inflammatory arthritis such as rheumatoid disease. It may be caused by the disease itself or by bleeding, or may be due to lack of haematinics such as iron, folate or B12. Sometimes it is caused by increased destruction of red cells as in Felty's syndrome when it is known as haemolytic anaemia. Because anaemia may be due to a number of different causes, the laboratory also report on the size and colour of red cells, as well as the haemoglobin concentration. This report may be descriptive or in figures. Normally appearing red cells are described as being normochromic (ie having a normal colour) and normocytic (ie a normal size and shape). The red cells normally appear like this in rheumatoid anaemia. Red cells from a patient with iron deficient anaemia are typically pale coloured, ie hypochromic, and small, ie microcytic, whilst in B12 and folate deficiency they are macrocytic (large). The size of the red cells can also be expressed numerically as the mean corpuscular volume (MCV) and the amount of haemoglobin in the red cells, as the mean corpuscular haemoglobin or the mean corpuscular haemoglobin concentration.

White cell count. Normal values are from 5 to 10 000 per cu mm. The white cells in the blood comprise several types: neutrophil, eosinophil and basophil granulocytes, and lymphocytes and monocytes. Either the total white cell count or one type of white cell may be affected by diseases or drugs. For example, infections and the administration of steroids both result in a high neutrophil cell count. Polyarteritis nodosa is often associated with a high eosinophil count and drugs such as gold and penicillamine may cause depression of the total white cell count.

Platelets. Normal values are from 200 to 500 000 per cu mm. Platelets are small blood cells essential for the normal clotting process. Like the white cells they may be affected by rheumatic diseases or by drugs. A decrease of platelets is known as thrombocytopenia and is something which is particularly watched for in drug reactions especially to gold, penicillamine and cytotoxic drugs such as azathioprine. It is because these anti-rheumatic drugs are so prone to affect the blood count that when they are administered a careful eye is kept on the haemoglobin concentration, white cell count and platelet numbers.

Serum iron concentration. Serum iron concentration is low in rheumatoid arthritis and as a rule it is not because the patient is short of iron. Iron in the blood is carried on a protein and the capacity for carrying iron can be measured and expressed as the iron binding capacity (IBC). If the body is short of iron there is spare carrying capacity and the IBC is raised. In active rheumatoid arthritis the IBC is low and this roughly correlates with activity of the disease.

Acute phase reactants. There are a number of changes that often take place in the constituents of the blood during illness. These changes can be measured and are referred to as acute phase reactants. Although not specific for any particular illness, they are sensitive to the activity and severity of the illness. The most well known of these measurements is the erythrocyte sedimentation rate or ESR (sometimes called the BSR). Other reactants sometimes measured are for example, C reactive protein, changes in plasma proteins and plasma viscosity. In many laboratories the plasma viscosity is now measured routinely instead of the ESR (normal value less than 1.72 cp).

ESR. The ESR measures how much the red cell corpuscles sink when blood is left standing. It is a measurement of great antiquity, and estimates of the ESR were made by the Ancient Greeks. The propensity of the red cells to sink is directly related to their tendency to clump together. These clumps are called rouleaux (Fig. 13. 1). In turn the main factor which affects rouleaux formation is the quantity of fibrinogen in the blood. The ESR is now commonly measured by the Westergren method. Blood after venipuncture is diluted with sodium citrate which prevents clotting, and placed in a hundred millimetre glass tube. After one hour the depth to which the red cells have sunk is measured and expressed in millimetres. The normal value for males is from 0 to 10 mm and females from

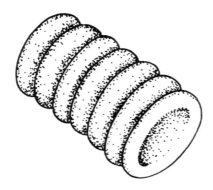

Fig. 13.1 Red cells in rouleaux formation.

0 to 15 mm. The contraceptive pill, menstruation, anaemia and pregnancy all result in false high values whilst false low results occur in congestive heart failure, sickle cell anaemia and polycythemia. Values also tend to be high in apparently well old people. The ESR is raised in most sorts of active illness, in particular, in inflammatory arthritis and collagen diseases, infections and neoplastic diseases. This is a good test for the presence of organic illness. The ESR is also used to monitor the effect of treatment, eg when treating rheumatoid arthritis with gold, or infections with antibiotics, recovery should be accompanied with a return towards normal of the ESR.

Biochemistry

Blood urea. Urea in the blood is derived from the breakdown of protein. The normal concentration is less than 40 mg/100 ml or 6.5 mmol/l. The kidneys are responsible for excreting it and a raised urea normally indicates renal disease. It may also occur however in dehydration, and when large quantities of protein are broken down suddenly in the gut, as in gastrointestinal haemorrhage.

Electrolytes. Serum sodium, potassium, chloride and bicarbonate are commonly measured in the blood. These are altered in many diseases. Diuretics and corticosteroids both decrease serum potassium.

Calcium and phosphorus. The normal plasma concentration is between 9 and 10.5 mg/100 ml and phosphorus between 3 and 4.5 mg/100 ml. Plasma calcium is low in hypoparathyroidism, osteomalacia and diseases where there is a low serum albumin, as in nephrotic syndrome. It is raised in hyperparathyroidism, vitamin D overdose, sarcoidosis and bone cancers. Plasma phosphorus tends to mirror calcium. These values vary at different times of the day and ideally blood calcium and phosphorus should be taken fasting and without a tourniquet.

Alkaline phosphatase. This is an enzyme produced by liver, intestine and bone. The normal value is less than 13 King Armstrong units per 100 ml. Bone alkaline phosphatase is raised during the healing of fractures, in osteomalacia and rickets, and is also raised, sometimes very greatly in Paget's disease of bone. It is an indication of bone formation. The liver enzyme is raised in obstructive jaundice and in tumours and inflammation of the liver. If necessary the enzymes from bone and liver can be distinguished biochemically.

Serum enzymes. Enzymes other than alkaline phosphatase can be measured in the blood. These enzymes are released from the cells which contain them when there is tissue damage.

Serum glutamic oxaloacetic transaminase and serum glutamic pyruvate transaminase (SGOT, SGPT). These enzymes are present in liver and muscle including heart muscle and are normally below 40 and 35 units per millilitre respectively. They are increased in muscle disease, liver disease and following myocardial infarction.

LACTATE DEHYDROGENASE (LDH). This enzyme is raised in the same diseases that increase the transaminases. The normal value is less than 500 units per millilitre.

CREATINE PHOSPHOKINASE (CPK) AND ALDOLASE. These enzymes are particularly useful in diagnosing and monitoring inflammation and other diseases of muscles. CPK is also raised after myocardial infarction. It should also be noted that the CPK may also increase after intramuscular injections and a mis–diagnosis of muscle disease could be made in this way.

Liver function tests. As well as measuring the above enzymes, ie alkaline phosphatase, transaminases and LDH which increase in liver disease, the serum bilirubin gives an indication of the liver function. Bilirubin is formed from the breakdown of haemoglobin and is normally excreted by the liver via the biliary system. Obstruction of the biliary ducts by gall stones, cancer or inflammation of the liver blocks the excretion and bilirubin accumulates in the blood. If great enough, clinical jaundice results. Excessive bilirubin may also be produced when excessive destruction of red cells (haemolysis) occurs.

Serum proteins and flocculation tests. In severe chronic liver disease serum albumin is reduced and globulin increased. Some laboratories also use non-specific tests for serum protein abnormality as an indication of liver disease, eg thymol and zinc sulphate turbidity tests.

MEASUREMENT OF SERUM PROTEINS. Serum proteins may be separated and measured by a method known as electrophoresis. In this method molecules with different electrical charges separate out on a strip, usually made of cellulose acetate. After staining, the different proteins can be demonstrated (Fig. 13.2). These different proteins have

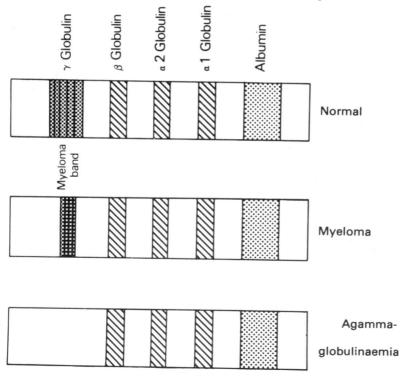

Fig. 13.2 Serum protein electrophoresis strips showing examples of three patterns: normal, myeloma and agammaglobulinaemia.

been labelled albumen, alpha 1, alpha 2, beta and gamma globulin. These constituents can be quantified if necessary. Serum protein electrophoresis is important in the diagnosis of myeloma, where the malignant plasma cells produce a very discrete protein which shows up as a definite band known as an M band on the electrophoretic strip. One type of arthritis is associated with low or absent gamma globulin.

IMMUNOGLOBULINS (IG). Serum proteins which carry antibodies can also be measured using an immunological technique in which the proteins are characterized as IgG, A, M, D and E. These immunoglobulin classes serve different functions and have different properties. In practice usually only IgG, IgA and IgM are measured.

Serum uric acid. The level of uric acid in the blood is a function of the amount produced by the body and the ability of the kidneys to get rid of it. The normal level is less than 7 mg/100 ml (0.42 mmol per litre) for men and 5 mg/100 ml for women. Concentration is almost always raised in people with gout which is caused by the deposition of urate crystals in the joints. The serum uric acid is raised in kidney disease and the blood urea should always be measured with the serum uric acid.

Biochemical measurements of urine. Many of the substances measured in the blood can be profitably measured in the urine. Measurement of creatinine in the urine together with simultaneous blood measurements gives an indication of renal function known as clearance. Measurements of urinary calcium may be useful in bone disease and measurements of urinary uric acid will indicate whether hyperuricaemia is due to too much uric acid being made or not enough being excreted.

   The most useful urine test is a test for excess urinary protein. This may be performed in the usual way with a random sample of urine using proprietary dipstick methods such as labstix. The result can be expressed as milligrams per 100 ml or in grams per litre. If present a 24-hour urinary protein estimation should be made to estimate how much protein is being lost. The upper limit of normal is 40 mg in 24 hours. Continued loss of large amounts of protein, more than 3 grams a day, may result in a lowered serum albumin level and the onset of a nephrotic syndrome. Any renal disease can cause proteinuria. Toxicity of drugs such as penicillamine and gold are the commonest causes of slight and heavy proteinuria in rheumatological practice. However, renal amyloidosis in rheumatoid arthritis and the nephritis of SLE can both cause a nephrotic syndrome. Small amounts of proteinuria may be caused by these conditions, by urinary tract infections and by contaminated specimens particularly during menstruation. In myelomatosis, proteinuria of a special kind known as Bence Jones proteinuria occurs. This is due to the abnormal protein produced by the malignant myeloma cells and characteristically appears and disappears on heating the urine.

Immunology

Several rheumatic diseases are associated with abnormalities of immunity. The immune system is responsible for protecting the individual against infections and toxins. One method of doing this is by the production of proteins known as antibodies which neutralize the noxious agent. Antibodies are produced by plasma cells which derive from one type of lymphocyte. The production of antibodies is stimulated by the presence of this noxious agent whether it be microbe or toxin. The process is utilized in vaccination or immunization against infectious diseases like diphtheria, tetanus and poliomyelitis.

In several diseases abnormal antibodies are produced. These may be stimulated by and act against the body's own tissue instead of against exogenous matter. These antibodies are known as autoantibodies. In many diseases these autoantibodies are probably just byproducts of tissue damage but in some like SLE and rheumatoid arthritis, they appear to have an important role in producing disease. The detection of these autoantibodies is important in the diagnosis of disease and different types of antibody are associated with different diseases.

Rheumatoid factor. Rheumatoid factor is an antibody that the body produces against its own globulin. It is found in the blood in several chronic inflammatory states, eg tuberculosis, syphilis and bacterial endocarditis, as well as in rheumatoid arthritis. It is also detected in about 5% of the normal population, particularly old people. It is commoner amongst relatives of people with rheumatoid arthritis. As a rule people with rheumatoid factor positive rheumatoid arthritis do worse than those with rheumatoid negative rheumatoid arthritis. There are a number of ways of detecting rheumatoid factor. Two are commonly used: the Latex test and the sheep cell agglutination test, sometimes called the SCAT test or Rose Waaler test after the people who invented it. In the Latex test, the patient's serum is added to globulin–coated latex particles. If the serum contains rheumatoid factor the particles clump and the test is positive. In the SCAT test the serum is added to globulin–coated sheep cells. The Latex test is more sensitive and the SCAT more specific for rheumatoid arthritis. The result may be expressed in a titre. This is a method of describing how strongly positive the test is and is expressed in doubling fractions, eg 1:10, 1:20, 1:40, 1:80, 1:160, 1:320 etc. The higher the titre the more positive the result.

Antinuclear antibodies. Antibodies to the nuclei of cells are also detected in the blood of patients with rheumatic diseases, in particular SLE.

ANTINUCLEAR ANTIBODY (ANA OR ANF) In this test sections of rat liver are placed on a slide and then covered with serum from the patient. If antibodies are present to nucleii, these will bind to the nucleii of the rat liver cells and can be demonstrated by special techniques which make the antibody fluoresce when viewed under a microscope. If positive the patient is said to have antinuclear antibodies in the blood. The result can be titred as in rheumatoid factor and a quantified result obtained, eg ANA positive to a titre of 1:40. Positive ANA is found in many diseases, eg SLE, rheumatoid arthritis, scleroderma, myositis, liver disease, burns, and it may be secondary to drug treatment such as hydrallazine and anti–epileptic drugs. The antinuclear antibodies may be reported as having different patterns, eg homogenous and speckled. Different patterns are characteristic of different diseases.

LUPUS ERYTHEMATOSUS CELL (LE CELL). This was the first test in routine use to detect antinuclear antibodies. The patient's blood is shaken in a container with glass beads to damage white cells. Nuclear material from the damaged cells is attacked by antinuclear antibodies if they are present in the blood and the nuclear antigen/antibody complex is then engulfed by undamaged white cells. These engulfing white blood cells are known as LE cells and their presence is a good indication of the presence of antinuclear antibody.

ANTI–DNA ANTIBODIES. Antibodies to the DNA (deoxyribonucleic acid) component of the cell nucleus are specific for SLE and a high titre implies SLE nephritis.

Complement. This is a substance made up of a number of components which circulate in the blood. When an antigen attacks an antibody, the antigen antibody complex activates complement. Activated complement is necessary to produce an inflammatory reaction. For example, a bacterium is attacked by an antibody which binds to it. This reaction activates complement which is then responsible for attracting white cells to the bacteria and facilitating the engulfing of the bacteria by the white blood cell. In these reactions complement is used up. It follows, therefore, that low levels of complement suggest continuing antigen/antibody reactions. In SLE nephritis such a process is the cause of the kidney damage and measuring complement gives some idea of the success or otherwise of treatment. A low level suggests continuing damage and a return to normal levels suggests cessation of disease. Complement is usually measured as the CH 50 which is a measure of total complement or more often, some of its components are measured, eg the third and fourth components (C3 and C4).

Antistreptolysin titre. Infection with streptococcal bacteria results in the formation of antistreptococcal antibodies which circulate in the blood. One of these, the antistreptolysin antibody can be measured and is expressed as an antistreptolysin titre. This is important in the diagnosis of rheumatic fever which is caused by an abnormal reaction of the body to a streptococcal infection, and a raised ASOT is evidence of recent streptococcal infection.

Tissue typing. Tissue typing was developed to prevent organ transplant rejection. If organ and recipient are matched for tissue type as well as blood group, this improves the chance of organ survival. A person's tissue type is characterized by the possession of substances known as human leucocyte antigens on the exterior of white cells in much the same way that AB blood groups are carried on red cells. Each individual has up to four of these antigens. The importance of tissue typing to arthritis is that an individual's tissue type is controlled by specific genes. If a disease is associated with a high prevalence of one particular tissue type, it means that genetic factors are very important in its cause. It also implies that unaffected people with that particular tissue type are more likely to develop the associated disease given the right circumstances. Some examples of tissue type and disease association are as follows: ankylosing spondylitis and Reiter's disease are associated with tissue type HLA B27;

psoriasis vulgaris is associated with HLA B13 and BW17; juvenile diabetes with B8 and BW15.

Examination of synovial fluid

Aspiration of joints may be made for diagnostic purposes. Examination of synovial fluid will distinguish between inflammatory and non-inflammatory arthritis. Examination of the fluid for bacteria in suspected infection is essential and the finding of crystals of urate or pyrophosphate will clinch the diagnosis of gout or pseudogout respectively. Blood may be found in a joint in spontaneous haemarthrosis such as occurs in osteoarthritis and rheumatoid arthritis, in villo-nodular synovitis and in bleeding diseases like haemophilia.

The normal appearance of synovial fluid is a clear, light straw coloured fluid. It is very viscous and when allowed to drop from the end of a needle will form a long string. Inflammation of a joint causes the fluid to become much less viscous and more cloudy according to the number of cells in the fluid.

Mucin clot test. The addition of dilute acetic acid to synovial fluid produces a thick white clot. The tighter the clot the less inflammatory the fluid, whereas in the presence of severe inflammatory arthritis such as active rheumatoid arthritis, the clot will not form properly at all and is then described as a 'poor mucin clot'.

Synovial fluid protein. Normal synovial fluid contains 2 grams or less per 100 ml of protein. The higher the protein content the more inflammatory the fluid.

Cells. Synovial fluid with little inflammation contains few white cells and conversely synovial fluids from patients with active rheumatoid arthritis or gout will contain high numbers of white cells in the fluid. In active inflammation the cells are predominantly polymorphonuclear and leucocytes. In early rheumatoid arthritis the cells are predominantly mononuclear cells.

Crystals. Crystals are looked for using polarized light which makes the crystals shine against a black background when viewed through a microscope. Urate crystals can be distinguished from calcium pyrophosphate crystals by the different shapes, and by the fact that they bend the polarized light in a different fashion. Other crystals such as those of cholesterol may also be seen in synovial fluid.

Synovial fluid is examined in the usual way for infection, particularly by direct staining and by culture techniques.

14
Drugs in Rheumatology

Drugs play an important part in the treatment of rheumatic diseases. Anti-rheumatic drugs are given to reduce pain and inflammation and in some cases suppress or influence the course of the disease.

A wide variety of drugs other than anti-rheumatic drugs may be used in rheumatic patients as of course they may often have diseases apart from their rheumatism. However, in this chapter we will deal only with those drugs used most often by the rheumatologist. Unfortunately, many drugs have serious unwanted side effects and it is therefore pertinent to those dealing with rheumatic patients that they have a broad knowledge of the possible consequences of treatment. It is especially true of the nurse who in hospital is in the most constant contact with the patient and is in a position thereby, to detect the earliest sign of a toxic effect. Nurses are also responsible for the administration of drugs which may be causing the patient's symptoms. If a nurse suspects that a patient may be suffering from the side effects of a particular drug, it is essential that she contacts the doctor responsible for the prescription as soon as possible and withholds the drug.

Drugs usually have at least two names, the approved or generic name and the proprietary or brand name which is given by the manufacturer; for example, indomethacin is the approved or generic name and Indocid the brand or proprietary name. If a compound is sold by several pharmaceutical companies it may have as many brand names. For example, penicillamine is sold by two drug companies and there are, therefore, two brand names, Distamine and Depamine. Whenever possible the approved name should be used.

Most anti-rheumatic drugs are given by mouth. Although food hinders the absorption of drugs by the gut it is common practice to give anti-rheumatic drugs at meal times in order to reduce the indigestion that they are prone to cause. Absorption of drugs can also be affected by the coating of the tablet; for example, the enteric coating of aspirin tablets may prevent the tablet breaking down in the gut, thereby preventing absorption.

Some drugs are given last thing at night to reduce morning stiffness on waking. These may be given by rectal suppository just before the patient retires. It is important that the patient knows what the suppositories are for, ie for morning symptoms and not for 'the bowels' and the nurse should make sure that the patient knows how, and is able, to insert them.

We are very much aware these days of drug interaction, ie the actions of different drugs clashing in the body. Anti-rheumatic drugs of the aspirin type may interfere with anti-coagulant drugs and produce local bleeding and make the anti-coagulant drug difficult to control.

Pain is the predominant symptom in arthritis and even inert and inactive tablets may abolish it by what is known as a *placebo* reaction (Latin placere—to please). About 50% of people may respond to placebo tablets in this way. One of the uses of a clinical trial is to decide whether the effect of a drug is due to its pharmacological properties or due to a placebo effect.

Clinical trials

To determine a drug's usefulness it is necessary to conduct what are known as clinical trials where the drug is tested for efficacy and toxicity. A clinical trial is any situation where the treatment to be tested is given in a predetermined way and the effects of the treatment are measured and recorded. A clinical trial should always incorporate a control with which the treated patient is compared, eg a patient's pre-treatment ESR can be compared to his ESR after five months of gold treatment. A fall in the ESR after such treatment would suggest that the gold had been effective. In this case the patient acts as his own control. Alternatively the treatment could be judged by comparing the treated patient with a similar but untreated patient. In this case it is the untreated patient who is the control.

In broad terms there are two types of clinical trial, open and blind. In an open trial the patient and doctor are both aware of what treatment has been prescribed. Open trials are very useful in the early stages of drug development when animal experiments have been completed and the drug is being cautiously tried out on a few people. Open trials are also used later on when the drug is being tried out on large numbers of people for a long time in order to assess unwanted effects. The disadvantage of open trials is that the doctor and patient may be biased against or in favour of the treatment to be tested and unconsciously influence the results. To overcome this prejudice, the blind trial was devised. In the blind trial either doctor or patient or both do not know the nature of the treatment that the patient is taking. When either doctor or patient is unaware of the treatment the trial is known as a single blind trial and when both do not know, the trial is known as a double blind trial. At the end of the trial the nature of the drugs administered is revealed and an unbiased conclusion can be drawn as to the drug's efficacy.

Blind trials are used to compare a test drug with a placebo and to compare a test drug with agents of known potency such as aspirin.

Classification and types of drugs

1. *Analgesics* (Table 14.1)

Analgesics are drugs that relieve pain and they vary from mild 'pain killers' such as paracetamol to very strong analgesics such as morphine. Some analgesics such as aspirin also reduce inflammation and these anti-inflammatory analgesics are considered in the next section.

Paracetamol is commonly used to kill the pain of osteoarthrosis. It is not suitable for rheumatoid arthritis as it does not reduce inflammation. It is given in a dose of one gram four times a day. In therapeutic doses it rarely causes side effects. Unfortunately, quite small amounts (20 tablets) can cause severe and sometimes fatal liver damage when used in non-accidental self-poisoning. Another drug commonly used in this class is dextropropoxyphene. It is commonly combined with other drugs, eg paracetamol, this combination being called Distalgesic. In many ways it is similar to codeine. For more severe pain pentazocine or dihydrocodeine (DF 118) may be used although both these drugs can cause nausea and drowsiness. It is most unusual for arthritics to require opiates, eg pethidine, but these may very occasionally be necessary.

2. *Drugs used to suppress inflammation and kill pain* (anti-inflammatory analgesics) (Table 14.2)

Aspirin. Aspirin or acetylsalicylic acid has been used as an anti-rheumatic drug for centuries. It was first obtained from the bark of a willow tree (*Salix*) hence its name. It was first synthesized in 1890 by the Bayer Company who called the product aspirin and this is now the approved name. It acts as an analgesic, ie a 'pain killer', and if given in sufficient quantities will also suppress the swelling and heat of inflamed joints in rheumatoid arthritis and other conditions. Aspirin probably works by preventing the production of prostaglandins which are substances important in the production of pain and

Table 14.1 Analgesics

Generic name	Proprietary name	Side effects	Formulation
Paracetamol	Panadol	Liver damage in large doses	Tablets 500 mg, 2 four hourly
Dextropropoxyphene	Distalgesic	Respiratory suppression in large doses	Tablets: DP 32.5 mg, paracetamol 325 mg 1 or 2 four hourly
Dihydrocodeine	DF 118	Constipation, especially in the elderly Drowsiness Lightheadedness Respiratory suppression in large doses	Tablets 30 mg, 1 or 2, 4–6 hourly Injections 50 mg, i.m.
Pentazocine	Fortral	Nausea, lightheadedness Respiratory suppression in large doses	Tablets 25 mg Caps. 50 mg 25–50 mg, 4–6 hourly Injection 30–60 mg, i.m.

There are many other preparations listed in MIMS, many of which contain combination of different analgesics, eg Paracodal (paracetamol and codeine), Veganin (aspirin, paracetamol and codeine).
Some contain tranquillizers, eg Equaprin (meprobamate and aspirin), and others caffeine eg Paralgin (paracetamol, caffeine and codeine).

Table 14.2 Anti-inflammatory Analgesics

Generic name	Proprietary name	Side effects*	Formulation
Aspirin	Aspirin	Tinnitus Dyspepsia. G.I.bleeding	Tablets 300 mg
Soluble aspirin Enteric-coated aspirin Benorylate	Disprin (and others) Nuseals Benoral	As for aspirin As for aspirin As for aspirin	Tablets 300 mg Tablets 300 & 600 mg Liquid 2 g in 5 ml
Indomethacin	Indocid	Peptic ulcer Headaches Mental confusion	Capsules 25 & 50 mg Suppository 100 mg
Phenylbutazone	Butazolidine	Aplastic anaemia Leucopenia Thrombocytopenia Rash Peptic ulcer	Tablets 100 mg
Oxyphenbutazone	Tanderil	As for phenylbutazone	Tablets 100 mg
Ibuprofen	Brufen	Dyspepsia	Tablets 200 & 400 mg
Ketoprofen	Orudis Alrheumat	Dyspepsia	Capsules 50 mg
Naproxen	Naprosyn	Dyspepsia	Tablets 250 mg
Fenoprofen	Fenopron	Dyspepsia	Capsules 300 mg

Other similar compounds are feprazone (Methrazone), sulindac (Clinoril), flufenamic acid (Arlef), mefenamic acid (Ponstan), fluclofenac (Flenac), flurbiprofen (Froben), and piroxicam (Feldene).

*All may cause indigestion and gastric bleeding, some are worse than others.

inflammation. The main drawback with aspirin is the number of unwanted side effects which cause withdrawal in 30% of patients. Aspirin frequently causes dyspepsia and clinically unnoticed gastric bleeding is common. Sometimes, however, massive bleeding may result from superficial gastric ulcers and require blood transfusion and surgery to save life. Because of these side effects it is unwise to take alcohol and aspirin together, to mix aspirin with drugs which inhibit clotting, eg anti-coagulants and to give aspirin to patients with a history of dyspepsia and peptic ulceration. It also causes tinnitus and in the elderly and children confusion and abnormal behaviour. Aspirin, because of its common use, is a source of accidental self-poisoning particularly among children. Aspirin is also a rare cause of urticaria and asthma. Despite these side effects, it must be remembered that massive amounts of aspirin are consumed yearly, about 2000 tons in the UK, most of which is bought over the chemist's counter which testifies that the public obviously regard it as a safe and efficacious remedy.

To overcome these side effects, various formulations have been tried. Soluble aspirin (Disprin) dissolves in water and is more rapidly absorbed and causes less gastric irritation. Aspirin coated to prevent dissolution in the stomach, for example, enteric-coated aspirin (Nuseals) lessens gastric irritation but absorption of the drug is uncertain as the enteric coating may not dissolve in time and the tablet may pass intact through the gut. This disadvantage can be detected if salicylate levels are measured in the blood after tablet consumption. A new form of aspirin medication is a combination of aspirin and paracetamol in liquid form and this liquid (benorylate) causes less gastric irritation but tinnitus is common.

As a 'pain killer' for use in osteoarthrosis, eight 300 mg tablets a day is the usual necessary dose. For suppression of joint inflammation as in rheumatoid arthritis, the dose is from twelve to sixteen 300 mg tablets daily (3.6 g to 4.8 g). In the child with arthritis 90 mg per kilogram body weight per day is a reasonable starting dose.

Over the years, many alternative drugs to aspirin have been manufactured in an attempt to obtain its analgesic and anti-inflammatory effects without its side effects. These are now commonly used in place of aspirin.

Indomethacin. Indomethacin (25 mg and 50 mg' capsules) is an effective analgesic and anti-inflammatory drug. It is given by mouth in capsule form in a dose of 75 mg to 150 mg per day and at night by suppositories (100 mg). It is liable to cause headaches, depression and confusion as well as peptic ulceration and gastrointestinal bleeding. The suppository may cause ano-rectal irritation.

Phenylbutazone. Phenylbutazone (100 mg) is a very effective anti-inflammatory drug. It is given by mouth and the dose should not exceed 300 mg per day if given for more than a week. It too tends to produce gastrointestinal bleeding and peptic ulceration. In addition, bone marrow depression causing thrombocytopenia (low levels of blood platelets which results in easy bruising and purpura), leucopenia (low white blood counts which causes low resistance to infection) and anaemia may occur. These toxic effects may be irreversible and fatal and it is the commonest drug to suppress bone marrow. It is particularly useful in the treatment of gout and ankylosing spondylitis but its toxicity restricts its use.

Ibuprofen, naproxen, ketoprofen, fenoprofen, flurbiprofen and others (see Table 14.2) are more recently synthesized compounds in use today, designed to decrease side effects without loss of efficacy. So far those drugs which give less trouble do seem to be less effective but do provide valuable alternatives for individual patients.

3. *Corticosteroids* (Table 14.3)

The cortisone family of drugs, often described just as steroids for short, is a group of very powerful anti-inflammatory agents. Hydrocortisone or cortisol is produced by the adrenal gland and is essential for life. It has been manufactured and can be used pharmacologically. Cortisone is very similar to cortisol. Its main effects are as follows: it causes the kidneys to retain salt and water; it increases the blood sugar, breaks down body protein and increases body fat on the trunk and face; it may cause peptic ulceration; it decreases the inflammatory response. It is this last property which makes it useful in patients with rheumatic disease. However, the unwanted side effects may be serious and include hypertension, diabetes mellitus, thin skin with the formation of striae and thin bones with a tendency to fracture, moon face, dyspepsia and gastrointestinal bleeding. The decrease in the inflammatory response although useful in some painful inflamed joints also decreases the resistance to infection, for example, old healed tuberculosis may start up again.

In an attempt to reduce side effects and to concentrate on the anti-inflammatory benefits, other types of steroids have been synthesized; the commonest used is prednisolone which is five times as

Table 14.3 Corticosteroids

Generic name	Proprietary name	Side effects	Formulation
Prednisolone		Dyspepsia Peptic ulcer Osteoporosis Diabetes mellitus Moon face Susceptibility to infection Pituitary suppression	Tablets 1 & 5 mg
Enteric-coated prednisolone	Delta Cortril	As above	Tablets 2.5 & 5 mg
ACTH preparations:			
Tetracosactrin injection	Synacthen & others	More tendency for hypertension	Injection 1 mg/ml
Corticotrophin injection	Acthar gel & others		Injection 20, 40 & 80 i.u./ml
Local Depot Preparations for Intra-articular Injections			
Hydrocortisone acetate	Hydrocortistab	Local infections Possible joint damage with frequent injections	Injection 25 mg/ml
Methylprednisolone Acetate	Depomedrone	As above	Injection 40 mg/ml
Triamcinilone		As above	Injection 20, 40 mg/ml

potent as cortisone in suppressing inflammation but causes less salt retention and, therefore, a lesser tendency to high blood pressure. Prednisone acts similarly but needs to be converted into prednisolone by the liver before it can work. Other even more potent anti-inflammatory steroids are methyl prednisolone, dexamethasone, betamethasone and triamcinolone.

Steroids may be given by mouth, by intra-muscular or intra-venous injection. They may also be given into joints as hydrocortisone acetate or methylprednisolone. If dyspepsia proves a problem with the oral route, enteric-coated prednisolone may be given. The risk of infection after injection with intra-articular steroids can be minimized by a scrupulous no-touch technique. Increasing pain or swelling after an intra-articular injection of steroid into a joint should always be reported immediately to a senior member of staff or to the doctor who gave the injection.

One of the most important side effects of steroid treatment is the suppression of the pituitary gland's production of adrenocorticotrophin (ACTH) and the resulting atrophy and inability of the body's own adrenals to produce cortisol in response to stress, eg accident, infection or surgical operation. For this reason steroid users should always be given extra steroids to cover any stress. Failure to do this may result in sudden collapse with low blood pressure and sometimes death. It is important that patients are aware of this risk and carry identification. It is equally important that any person concerned with their health care should realize the risk especially in the presence of a deteriorating patient. In an attempt to avoid this risk steroid treatment is sometimes given as ACTH injections either daily or less often. In this situation the ACTH stimulates the body's own adrenals to produce the extra steroid thus avoiding adrenal suppression. This treatment carries the disadvantage of unselective cortisol effect and the necessity of repeated injections.

The contribution of the nurse to the well-being of patients on steroids can be summed up as follows:

Blood pressure should be noted and reported if high or unduly low.
Urine should be tested for sugar.
A watch should be kept for stomach upset or passing of blood or a melaena stool.
A history of tuberculosis or other infection should be pointed out to the medical staff.
The patient should be informed of the necessity of regular

consumption of steroids. He should be given a steroid card and should be told the risks before going home.

Any joint deterioration after intra-articular steroid injection should be reported.

Finally make sure that steroid cover is prescribed and given if a patient who is a steroid user is going to have a surgical operation.

4. Drugs which cause a remission in rheumatoid arthritis (Table 14.4)

Chloroquine, gold, penicillamine, levamisole and immuno-suppressive drugs are drugs used mainly to suppress rheumatoid arthritis. In addition, chloroquine is also used for the treatment of systemic lupus erythematosus. They all have in common the fact that there is a delay of one to three months between the first administration of the drug and the onset of action. This is important as patients may become discouraged by the apparent lack of response to the medication and may discontinue the treatment prematurely.

Chloroquine. Chloroquine is a drug developed and used for the treatment of malaria. Chloroquine phosphate is given in a dose of 250 mg (1 tablet) per day for up to and not exceeding one year in the treatment of rheumatoid arthritis. Chloroquine sulphate (200 mg/day) or hydroxychloroquine (400 mg/day) are alternatives. The duration of the treatment is important as its most serious side effect, that of retinal damage, only occurs after one year of treatment (in fact it is rare before 550 g have been consumed). Other side effects are nausea, vomiting and rashes, and its deposition in the cornea of the eye causing the patient to see haloes around objects. Unlike the retinopathy these side effects are all easily reversible by stopping the drug. If it is thought desirable to continue treatment for more than twelve months, then regular ophthalmic examinations should be arranged.

Gold. Gold (sodium aurothiomalate, Myocrisin) may be very effective in suppressing the activity of rheumatoid arthritis and the benefit may be felt for a year or more after the course of gold has finished. Gold salts have to be given by intra-muscular injection. The usual practice is to give a 10 mg test dose followed by 50 mg, weekly for twenty weeks. Unwanted side effects are common and include suppression of the bone marrow, eg thrombocytopenia, leucopenia,

Table 14.4 Drugs which cause a Remission in Rheumatoid Arthritis

Generic name	Proprietary name	Side effects	Formulation
Chloroquine phosphate	Avloclor Resochin	Rash Nausea Eye damage after prolonged use	Tablets 250 mg 1 daily up to one year
Chloroquine sulphate	Nivaquine	As above	Tablets 200 mg 1 daily up to one year
Hydroxychloroquine	Plaquenil	As above	Tablets 200 mg 2 daily up to one year
Gold (sodium aurothiomalate)	Myocrisin	Rash Pruritus Renal damage Marrow suppression Diarrhoea Mouth ulcers	Injection i.m. 1, 5, 10, 20, 50 mg, amps
Penicillamine	Distamine Depamine	Rash Nausea Mouth ulcers Renal damage Marrow suppression Transient loss of taste	Tablets 50, 125, 250 mg

Generic name	Proprietary name	Side effects	Formulation
Levamisole		Nausea Skin rash Mouth ulcers Taste disturbance Tremors Marrow suppression	Tablets 50 mg
Azathioprine	Imuran	Nausea Dyspepsia Diarrhoea Marrow suppression	Tablets 50 mg
Cyclophosphamide	Endoxana	Nausea Dyspepsia Diarrhoea Marrow suppression Alopecia Cystitis	Tablets 50 mg

* Other immuno-suppressive drugs are very occasionally used in rheumatic diseases such as chlorambucil, methotrexate and melphalan.

skin rashes from simple itching to complete shedding of the epidermis, mouth ulcers, diarrhoea and toxic effects on the kidney producing proteinuria which if heavy may result in the nephrotic syndrome. Great care must therefore be taken in the use of gold and in some centres special Gold Clinics are set up. As it is often the nurse who administers gold injections, it is she who is most likely to first encounter side effects. Before each weekly injection, the patient should be questioned about itching or skin rash; the urine specimen should be checked for proteinuria; and the patient's blood should be checked for numbers of platelets, red blood cells and white cells. If this practice is followed, the risks are reduced to a minimum.

Penicillamine. Penicillamine is a substance that binds metals, particularly copper. It has been used in diseases other than rheumatoid arthritis for many years and in particular has been a mainstay in the treatment of Wilson's disease, in which excess amounts of copper are deposited in the brain and liver. Quite recently, it has been accepted as a useful alternative to gold in the treatment of rheumatoid arthritis. It comes in 50, 125 and 250 mg tablets and is taken by mouth. A low dose is used initially, the amount gradually being increased over a number of weeks. Its side effects are similar to those of gold: rashes, thrombocytopenia and proteinuria. In addition, it can cause nausea, dyspepsia and diarrhoea, mouth and tongue ulcers and occasionally loss of taste which is temporary.

As in the practice of gold administration, frequent checks of the patient's condition including urine and blood testing are essential. As the duration of the treatment lengthens these checks can be made less frequently but never less than three monthly.

Levamisole. Levamisole is a drug developed for the treatment of parasites such as roundworms. It has recently been found to have a beneficial effect in rheumatoid arthritis similar to that obtained with penicillamine.

Immuno-suppressive drugs (anti-cancer drugs). These drugs were developed initially for the treatment of cancer and are used to suppress tissue rejection after organ transplants, hence the term immuno-suppressive. They are now sometimes used in rheumatology particularly for the severe kidney disease of SLE and for patients with severe rheumatoid arthritis. They may produce a remission particularly in the latter condition. Drugs used most often are azathioprine (Imuran) and cyclophosphamide (Endoxana). These drugs may produce severe and unwanted side effects especially in the case of cyclophosphamide. The side effects include nausea, vomiting, diarrhoea, suppression of blood cell production causing anaemia, leucopenia, thrombocytopenia, and also in the case of cyclophosphamide, hair loss, cystitis and bladder fibrosis. There is also the theoretical risk of tumour induction. As with gold, although the possible side effects are daunting, if care with dosage and regular observation of the patient is practised, then these risks are minimized. Two further drugs recently used to induce remissions in RA are clozic and dapsone.

5. Drugs used in gout (Table 14.5)

Some drugs are used exclusively in gout. Colchicine is a drug extracted from the autumn crocus and has been used in medicine for thousands of years. It is still occasionally used in the treatment of the acute attacks of gout and as a prophylactic in preventing further attacks. Its main side effects are gastrointestinal. In the acute attack of gout, colchicine is used in a dose of 0.5 mg two hourly until the acute attack subsides or side effects, usually diarrhoea, supervene. The dose in prophylactic treatment is 0.5 mg, two or three times a day.

Probenecid is used to increase the excretion of urate from the kidneys thereby causing a fall in the serum uric acid. The dose used is 500 mg, three or four times a day. The main side effects are skin rashes and, as probenecid increases the excretion of uric acid, the formation of uric acid stones in the urinary tract (unless precautionary measures are taken).

Allopurinol interferes with the formation of uric acid in the body and thus reduces serum uric acid levels. The dose is 300 to 900 mg daily. Side effects are unusual but skin rashes may be troublesome.

6. Drugs, pregnancy and the fetus

Rheumatoid arthritis commonly affects young women, who may be expected to become pregnant. This fact should be remembered when drugs are prescribed for treatment. Drugs may affect the developing fetus and may, if excreted in the mother's milk, harm the newborn baby if breast fed. The safest policy is obviously to stop all drugs before conception takes place, but this is a council of perfection and rarely practical. Certainly the drugs used should be reduced to the minimum, well in advance of conception occurring. Some analgesic

Table 14.5 Drugs in Gout

Generic name	Proprietary name	Side effects	Formulation	Use
Colchicine		Nausea Dyspepsia Diarrhoea	Tablets 0.25 & 0.50 mg	Acute gout and prophylaxis
Probenecid	Benemid	Rashes Possible urinary calculi	Tablets 500 mg	Prevent gout by reducing the amount of uric acid in the body
Allopurinol	Zyloric	Rashes	Tablets 100 mg 300 mg	As above

drug will almost certainly need to be continued and aspirin is undoubtedly the safest. The effect on the fetus of the newer analgesic anti-inflammatory drugs is virtually unknown. Due to differences between animal species, the only way to find out the effect of a drug on a human fetus is to give it to a pregnant woman. Nowadays no one willingly does this and experience of such effects can only come by accident.

Of the more specific drugs for rheumatoid arthritis, chloroquine is known to be a hazard to the fetus. It is also excreted in breast milk and should not be given to mothers who are breast feeding.

Gold has possibly dangerous effects on the fetus. Penicillamine has been associated with the birth of abnormal children, though not in every patient taking penicillamine at the time of conception.

Azathioprine has never been definitely associated with an abnormal child and several normal children have been born to mothers taking it.

Cyclophosphamide is certainly dangerous to the fetus. Steroids can be continued in a dose of 7.5 to 10 mg a day, without ill effect.

Further Reading

Boyle, James. *Lecture Notes in Pharmacology and Therapeutics for Nurses*. Churchill Livingstone.

British National Formulary. British Medical Association and the Pharmaceutical Society of Great Britain. (Essential reading. Use this and not MIMS!)

Drug and Therapeutics Bulletin. The Consumer's Association. (For reference. Published fortnightly.)

Lawrence, D. R. *Clinical Pharmocology*, 4th edn. Churchill Livingstone. (The first few chapters on prescribing habits, experimentation and placebos are excellent value. For reference and entertainment.)

15
Physical Therapy

Although drug therapy is important in the treatment of all forms of arthritis, this has often to be supplemented by physical therapy. Physical therapy is designed to help reduce inflammation, prevent or correct deformities and maintain as full a range of movement as possible.

```
               Aims of Local Joint Treatment
    1. Reduce inflammation by resting joint
    2. Prevent deformity
    3. Correct deformity
    4. Maintain or improve power of surrounding muscles
    5. Maintain or increase range of movement at joint.
```

The physical methods that may be used include bed rest, splintage of joints, physiotherapy and hydrotherapy.

Rest

Rest of an inflamed joint is a fundamental principle of treatment of most forms of arthritis. This is often against the natural inclinations of the patient and his relatives. The symptom of early morning stiffness in joints which improves with exercise, suggests to the patient that such exercise is beneficial although in fact it increases damage to the joints. A frequent comment from patients is that they are afraid that they will 'seize up' if they do not continue to use their joints. However, it can be pointed out to patients that it is those joints which they use most often that are most inflamed. In right-handed people the right hand is usually more affected than the left. In hemiplegic patients with an inflammatory arthritis the paralysed side is much less severely affected than the normal.

Rest is relative. It can mean merely reducing a particular activity which over-uses a certain joint to complete bed rest for twenty-four hours a day. In between these two extremes rest may mean changing to lighter work, spending a period each day resting on the bed or using splints to support and prevent joints moving. Though the simplest advice to give to the patient, rest may be the most difficult part of the whole treatment programme to follow. The young housewife with children may find it very difficult to reduce her physical activity. Men who have to change jobs to 'lighter work' find always that this means less pay. Sometimes it has to be recognized that a substantial degree of rest is impossible, for example, the self-employed small shopkeeper or the busy accountant who may employ several people. However, it is our policy whenever possible to admit to hospital all early cases of inflammatory arthritis for a period of rest and assessment.

Prolonged bed rest in hospital may be associated with physical complications and emotional problems.

Physical Complications Associated with Prolonged Bed Rest

1. Joint contracture
2. Pressure sores
3. Deep vein thrombosis
4. Muscle wasting and 'bone wasting' ie osteoporosis
5. Difficulties with toileting and bathing

Physical Complications of Bed Rest. The difference between a 'good' bed position and a 'bad' bed position is the difference between good and bad nursing. In the good position there is a firm mattress sometimes with fracture boards as well, a firm angled back support, no pillows under the knees and the ankles protected from the weight of the bedclothes by a cage, sometimes supplemented by a foot board (Fig. 15.1).

Pressure sores are obviously likely in any patient on prolonged bed rest. In arthritis they may be made more likely by the difficulty and pain the patient suffers in changing position, perhaps in addition hampered by splints. Patients on steroids have thin skin that easily breaks down. Elderly patients living alone may have a dietary deficiency, particularly of vitamin C, which may also contribute to the rapid development of pressure sores. The presence of some or all of these factors may make healing of the sores difficult and secondary infection may spread from the bed sore to the blood stream and septicaemia and septic arthritis may follow. As always, prevention is easier than cure.

Deep vein thrombosis is common in patients immobilized in bed. However, arthritic patients rarely have such a thrombosis. This may

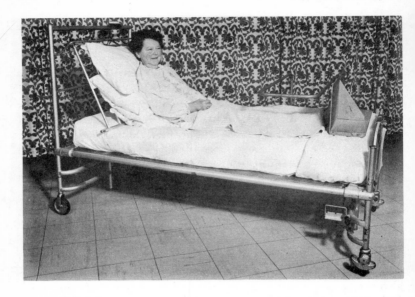

Fig. 15.1 Good bed position. Note fracture boards under mattress, firm back support, ankles protected by cradle and use of foot board.

be related to the analgesic drugs used which interfere with the stickiness of platelet cells in the blood and thus interfere with blood coagulation.

In any patient on prolonged bed rest wasting of the muscles occurs. In arthritis this is far greater than might be expected to follow from bed rest alone and seems partly to result from the arthritis in the adjacent joints. This wasting should be corrected as far as possible by exercises. Remember that the stability of many joints depends on the power of the surrounding muscles.

Wasting of bones also occurs with bed rest and although this is usually not important it may occasionally be severe, particularly in elderly patients who are on steroids. Exercises probably help to reduce the bone loss. In extreme cases renal stones may be formed from the large amount of calcium being excreted via the kidney.

Toileting and bathing. At first it seems reasonable to allow bed resting patients to walk to the toilet and back. Experience shows that a visit to the toilet may mean two half hourly chats with patients en route, collecting a bottle for another patient and a final half hour watching television in the day room! The alternative of providing bottles and bedpans for all bed resting patients is very demanding on nursing time and a reasonable compromise is to wheel patients to the bathroom and toilet in chairs.

Emotional Problems of Prolonged Bed Rest. Prolonged rest as used here, implies rest in a hospital bed. Satisfactory rest can rarely be obtained at home. Frequently we see patients who say that they have been resting at home without any marked improvement, but after only a few days of complete rest in hospital they feel much better. Complete bed rest in hospital means complete rest, no getting up to find some missing family necessity or just to watch television for a few minutes, etc.

The first emotional problem likely to occur after admission is a sense of isolation from other members of the family. Many patients with arthritis have marital problems (see Chapter 17) and an additional worry may be about the fidelity of the spouse left at home. Women with babies should, if possible, not be separated from them and our policy in these cases, where the mother needs admission, is also to take in the young child and keep them together in a side ward. Isolation can be reduced further by flexible visiting hours.

Patients with arthritis do better nursed away from acute wards. Acute wards are busy with frequent admissions, deaths and discharges. Nights may be noisy from emergency admissions and restless patients. A patient with arthritis will probably spend several weeks and occasionally several months in hospital; he needs peace and quiet and a tempo in which the unit of time is measured in days rather than hours, and weeks rather than days.

A further problem is the distress that the new patient faces on seeing advanced cases of arthritis in the ward. This may have some rewards for the patient. It allows him to see that even in advanced disease some form of treatment is possible. He has a chance to assess in his own mind the importance to his life style of his arthritis and it perhaps encourages him to follow medical advice in order to reduce joint damage to the minimum. Many patients find encouragement when they see that there are other patients like them and know that they are not an isolated case. This lessens the sense of injustice that some patients feel at having been 'picked on' by an unkindly fate.

If the patient's stay is to be as happy as possible as much attention needs to be paid to his emotional problems as to his pressure areas! The nurse needs to be aware of this and to be ready to establish a relationship with the patient and his relatives based on mutual trust and confidence. She must remember that not only the newly diagnosed patient has problems; the long-standing patient may be depressed, may be worried about financial problems or may have fears about his proposed treatment. Time spent talking to the patient should be regarded not as wasted but as an essential nursing duty. Patients may need repeated admissions and their willingness to 'come in' will be greatly influenced by the atmosphere on the ward. A good atmosphere does not just happen, it has to be worked at by all those members of staff, not only nurses, who work on the ward. Because the nurse comes into the closest and most prolonged contact with the patient, her influence is critical.

In the face of disability and loss of function, the constant emphasis has to be on what function is left rather than dwelling on that which has been lost. It has been said that it is not until the patient (and his family) is willing to 'let go' of the function that has been lost, can he (and his family!) move on to the next stage in a recovery programme.

Finally, let the nurse remember that she ill serves her patients if she overprotects them. At times the patient has to struggle, for example, in getting dressed or has to take the risk of falling when walking, if he is to gain confidence in himself and become more independent.

Emotional Problems of Prolonged Bed Rest
(in hospital)

1. Isolation from other members of the family, particularly children
2. Lack of quiet on 'acute' wards
3. The presence of other patients with more advanced disease

Splints

The original definition of a splint is a device for keeping fractured bones in position. Nowadays the word is used to cover a much broader series of appliances whose functions may be divided into rest, supportive and corrective roles. They may be made of plaster of Paris (POP), leather, plastic or metal.

Splints

1. Rest
2. Supportive
3. Corrective

Plaster of Paris splints are cheap, easy to make and require no special equipment but they do not wear well, are heavy and are not waterproof. POP splints are usually used, therefore, where splints have to be changed frequently and used for only a short period of time.

Plastic splints are available in a variety of materials. They all have the benefit of being light in weight, long lasting and waterproof but all have the disadvantage of needing heat for moulding and precise moulding is a skilful process. All are relatively expensive. Plastic splints are usually designed for longer term use and where cosmetic factors are important.

Leather splints are similar to plastic ones in that they are lighter than plaster of Paris and more durable but unlike plastic splints, they are not waterproof. They need considerable skill to make and are fairly expensive.

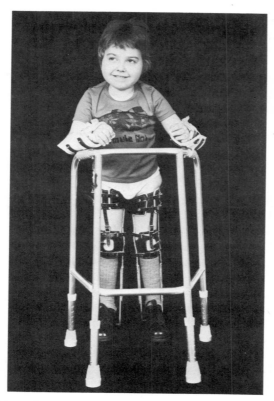

Fig. 15.2 Leg calipers used here in a young boy with severe Still's disease.

Metal splints are more difficult than plastic to shape; like plastic they are waterproof. They are used where greater strength is needed than plastic can supply, for example, in calipers for knees and ankles (Fig. 15.2).

All splints may damage underlying skin and all tend to cause muscle wasting around the splinted joint unless precautions are taken. If incorrectly fitted they may do more harm than good.

Rest splints. These are supplied to hold a joint in a fixed position. They are usually made of plaster of Paris and examples are shown in Figs. 15.3 to 15.6. It is important to note that each joint has an ideal rest position, in which the strain on the joint is minimal, pain is relieved and later function is protected.

Hands and wrists are supported with the wrist in 10–20° of extension and the fingers relaxed in a semi-flexed position (Fig. 15.3).

Elbows are supported at 90° of flexion with the hand midway between pronation and supination.

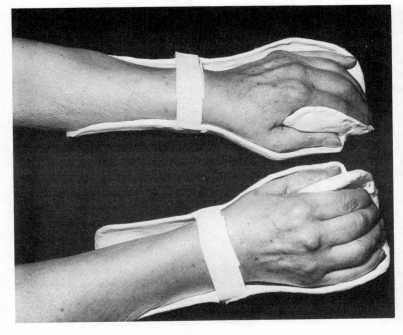

Fig. 15.3 Rest plasters for hands.

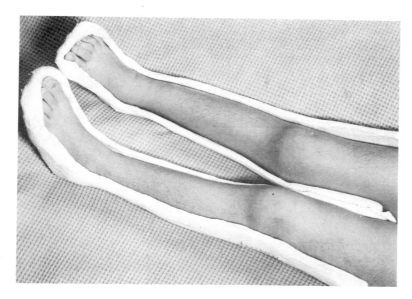

Fig. 15.5 Gutter leg splints.

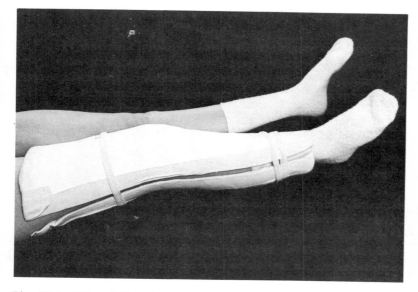

Fig. 15.4 'Hinged' POP knee splint. This can be removed for exercises, etc.

Ankles are supported in the neutral position, midway between dorsi and plantar flexion. It is particularly important to check this position as ankles are easily immobilized in some degree of plantar flexion and permanent disability due to contracture of the Achilles tendon can occur.

The knees should be splinted in maximum extension (Fig. 15.4).

Rest splints may be either a full plaster of Paris cylinder (the limb is completely encircled by the plaster) or of a partial shell or gutter design (Figs. 15.5 and 15.6). The full cylinder ensures that the patient cannot remove it! It also provides maximum support to the joint but does present problems with toileting and other forms of treatment such as hydrotherapy though static quadriceps exercises can still be carried out in a full POP splint. Gutter splints can be re-

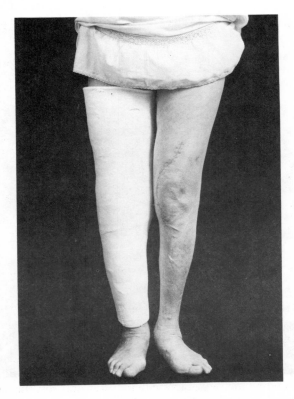

Fig. 15.6   Full knee cylinder used here to support the knee when walking.

moved easily (for better or worse!) and bathing and toileting are easier.

Supportive splints. These splints are designed to support the joint while it is being used. The commonest example is a polythene wrist splint (Fig. 15.7). Most splints in this group are made of various types of plastic.

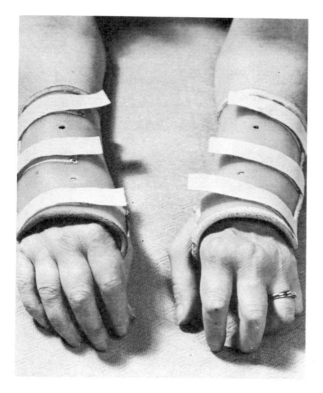

Fig. 15.7   Polythene wrist splints.

The cervical spine can be supported by a variety of collars, from simple cardboard to rigid polythene or blocked leather (Fig. 15.8). The lumbar and thoracic spine can also be splinted by a variety of supports. No form of spinal support is able to stop movement of the spine completely. Their use may help by providing warmth, partial support and reduction of movement. At times we suspect these supply more support to the mind than to the spine.

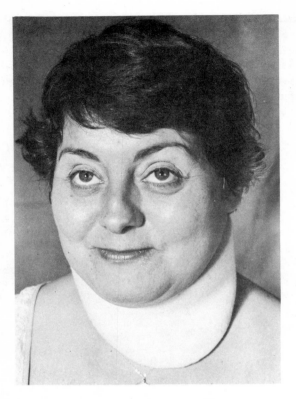

Fig. 15.8 Soft cervical collar (see also photograph, p. 54).

Calipers. Calipers were used extensively in the past but with improvements in surgery are less often used today. Perhaps the commonest use now is to support the ankle with either a 'double iron below knee caliper' or an 'outside iron and T strap caliper'.

Corrective splints. These are designed to correct joint deformity. The commonest type is probably a serial knee plaster. Here flexion deformity of the knee is corrected by applying a full cylinder plaster to the knee while at the same time putting pressure on the thigh and lower leg to straighten the knee. The plaster is changed after a few days and the process is repeated as often as necessary. With this technique quite severe, 45° or more, flexion deformity can often be corrected. Whether skin traction counts as a form of splinting, it is

certainly an effective alternative to serial plasters for flexion deformities of the knee. It is probably more uncomfortable and restricting
to the patient. Thin skin, which is common in rheumatoid arthritis,
may make the attachment of the skin traction an additional difficulty.
Leg traction may also be used to distract the hip and reduce rest pain
in hip joints.

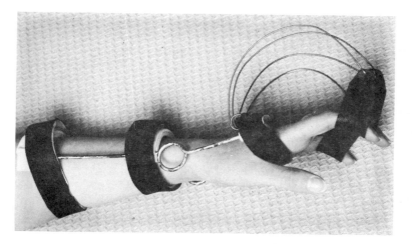

Fig. 15.9   Lively splint.

A special type of splint used after hand surgery is called a 'lively'
splint (Fig. 15.9). This offers partial support for the metacarpo-
phalangeal joints but movement at these joints is still possible pulling
against the resistance of elastic bands, or wire springs.

Exercise

It may seem strange having used a good deal of space to describe the
benefit of rest that we now discuss the place of exercise in the
treatment of arthritis. Exercises have two functions: (1) to maintain
or improve the power of muscles around the joints, and (2) to
maintain or improve the range of movement in the joint. Most of the
exercises belong to the field of the physiotherapist, although there is
some overlap with the work of the occupational therapist and
occasionally the craft therapist. Exercises may be passive or active. In
passive exercises the patient does not use his own muscles, the joint

being moved through its range by the therapist. Active exercises involve the patient using his own muscles. The force used to move the joints may be reduced by assisted movement where part of the force is supplied by slings or the assistance may be given by the support of water during hydrotherapy. With better muscle power exercises are carried out against the resistance of gravity or if greater resistance is needed, against weights or springs resisting joint movement. In general several short periods of exercises a day are better than one prolonged single session. Except in the most acutely inflamed joints (which are anyway probably being protected by splints) each joint should be put through its full range of movement once a day. The therapist starts with the mildest types of exercises and carefully assesses the effect on the joint. Any exacerbation of pain, swelling or early morning stiffness is a warning that the amount of exercise must be reduced.

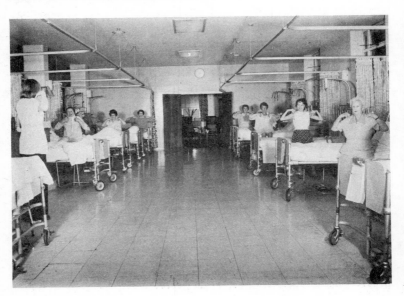

Fig. 15.10 Ward class.

Later, as the patient becomes more mobile, more specific 'functional' exercises can be commenced, eg walking, getting up off the floor, etc. When attempting to walk any disabled patient, not only those affected by disease of joints, it is important to remember that this must proceed from stage to stage and no attempt to move to the next stage should be made unless the present stage is satisfactory.

The first stage is for the patient to be able to sit upright on a stool, next to stand in balance using a support if necessary, next to stand on one leg, again using a support, and then and only then, to swing one leg through and to start walking. If you think about it you will see how impossible it is for someone who cannot stand to walk. Yet all too often one sees patients, perhaps with hemiplegia, being half dragged across the floor (terrifying to the patient) and the result called walking exercises. Far better to spend the time getting the patient to balance on two feet and gaining confidence in himself as he does so.

Pain when using the joint may be reduced by the prior application of either local heat, usually in the form of short wave diathermy, or ultrasound or oddly, cold. Which is better seems to vary from patient to patient and there is little place, in hospital practice, for these measures unless followed by exercises although the patient at home may find the local application of heat or cold to the joints soothing.

Hydrotherapy (therapeutic use of water). Although in the past the 'waters' were taken internally and used externally in a variety of contrast sprays, bubble baths, etc, nowadays hydrotherapy is virtually confined to pool therapy. The hydrotherapy pool is filled with

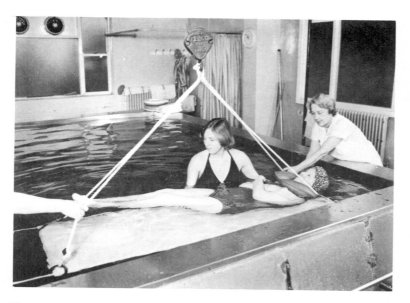

Fig. 15.11 Hydrotherapy pool.

water almost at body temperature. The precise chemical constitution of the water although given importance in the past, is today ignored and tap water is as good as any spa water. Water gives partial support to the joints and its warmth relaxes muscles and reduces pain.

In the pool, joints can be mobilized gently and put through a range of movement without strain. After a period of bed rest pool therapy is often used before weight bearing is commenced. Because of the fairly high temperature of the water it can be a fatiguing therapy for some patients and all patients need a period of rest after each treatment. Open wounds and incontinence of bladder or bowels are contra-indications to pool therapy but some POP splints can be protected in polythene bags to allow treatment.

Objects of Exercise

1. To maintain or improve muscle power
2. To maintain or improve range of joint movement
3. To help achieve functional target
   ie walking, climbing stairs, etc

Physical Methods of Pain Relief

Treatment by heat, cold and sound. The application of heat can be very soothing in arthritis. Pain is often relieved and joint stiffness and muscle spasm overcome. It is often conveniently used before exercises are begun. There are various ways of applying heat.

The wax bath for years has been a traditional method of applying heat to hands and feet. Similarly many people with arthritis find that immersing their hands in warm water relieves morning stiffness. Heat may also be applied by electrical means, such as the infra-red, short-wave and microwave systems.

Infra-red lamps produce the non-visible infra-red part of the light spectrum. When directed against part of the body, infra-red rays have a warming effect, although only the superficial tissues are warmed.

Short-wave diathermy is so called because the machine produces electromagnetic waves of short wave length (in contrast to the longer wave lengths of infra-red waves). Treatment is applied by placing the part to be treated between two condensor plates. When the machine is switched on an electric field is set up between the plates and the tissue within that field becomes warmed. This treatment is therefore the best method of applying heat to deep structures such as the hip. For technical reasons it is important to ensure that the patient has no metal, eg a fracture plate or prosthesis, in the treated part as this may induce a deep burn.

Microwave diathermy irradiates the tissues with waves intermediate between infra-red and short wave; similarly the depth of the heating is also intermediate.

The physiotherapist is trained to take the necessary precautions to make sure that overheating and burning do not take place. Nevertheless, it is wise to be aware that these treatments can produce burns and if the patient signals that the treatment is uncomfortable and becoming painful, the apparatus should be turned off.

In some circumstances the application of cold ice packs has a pain-relieving function and can be used as a pre-exercises treatment.

Ultrasound treatment consists of applying high frequency sound waves to tissues. It has found favour in the treatment of soft tissue lesions particularly in ligamentous tears and sport injuries.

Acupuncture. Acupuncture consists of the insertion of needles through the skin. Nerve endings are stimulated by twirling the needles or applying a small electric current to them. Needles are inserted in locations mapped out by Chinese physicians. Acupuncture probably results in transient analgesia and any benefit it has is limited by the short duration of its effect.

Hypnosis. Hypnosis has been used for thousands of years to treat illness. Various other techniques such as yoga and meditation probably have a similar end state, the production of a 'trance'. It seems that the mind exists in three states: awake, sleeping and 'trance'. Unfortunately scientific evidence that the trance state exists and is different to the waking state is lacking. The electro-encephalogram cannot distinguish between the two. This difficulty of deciding and defining the trance state has divided doctors over the centuries into those in favour and those against. Hypnosis in this country may be practised by doctors or lay persons.

The inducing of a hypnotic trance is not a difficult feat, though it may be slow. There is no doubt that some people under hypnosis are able to withstand what in other circumstances would be extreme pain, with apparent indifference. Fractured bones can be manipulated, wounds sutured, etc. while the patient seems completely relaxed.

It might seem therefore that hypnosis would be extremely useful for chronic painful illnesses such as arthritis. It is very unlikely that hypnosis could reduce the inflammation accompanying rheumatoid arthritis that is responsible in the first place for the pain.

The drawbacks to hypnosis are that few doctors are trained in its use and that it is still, in many minds, associated more with 'quackery' than proper medicine. Perhaps the biggest drawback, however, that has prevented further research into its effectiveness, is the time taken to induce a trance of sufficient depth to be effective and the uncertainty that such depth can be obtained regularly in a sufficient number of patients. Over the last twenty years there has been a gradual increase in interest in medical hypnosis and as mind and body continue to be found to be inseparable in diseased patients, hypnosis may yet emerge into routine medical practice. Probably, at least, hypnosis can do little harm to the patient.

16
Surgery

Surgery is not a cure for arthritis but its use at the right time can do much to help the arthritic patient. Close cooperation between the rheumatologist and the surgeon with an understanding of each other's role is important. With multiple joint involvement the state of the other joints may be the critical factor if success is to follow operation. For example, in surgery to the knee, the state of the other joints in the affected leg, hip, ankle and foot will determine how much mobility will follow operation. The state of the hands, for gripping a walking stick, and elbows and shoulders for providing partial weight bearing through walking sticks post-operatively needs to be considered. An operation on a hip that increases the patient's mobility may greatly accelerate deterioration in a knee and after a short interval the patient's mobility is reduced to its previous level, although now by knee pain and deformity. The domino effect of improvement in one joint throwing greater strain on the other joints needs to be considered constantly. Few operations are urgent and the decision whether to operate or not can be taken at leisure, sometimes after a period of medical treatment and observation in hospital. As always the patient's motivation is of prime importance and will often largely determine how much mobility the patient regains after surgery.

Soft Tissue Operations

1. Biopsy
2. Decompression
   Nerves
   Tendons
3. Tenotomy
4. Synovectomy

Soft Tissue Operations

Biopsy

Biopsy usually involves removing part of the synovium from a joint in order to aid the diagnosis. Its main use is in infective conditions, such as tuberculous arthritis and in the rare neoplastic growths within a joint. It is less helpful in trying to distinguish between the different types of inflammatory arthritis. A biopsy is also needed at times for lesions in bones, such as myeloma or secondary deposits from cancer elsewhere.

It is possible to inspect the inside of some joints through an arthroscope and a biopsy may be taken at the same time under direct vision. At the moment this is not a routine process and its value is being assessed.

Decompression of nerves and tendons

The soft tissue swelling that occurs in inflammatory arthritis quite commonly causes pressure on some nerves. The commonest site is pressure on the median nerve at the wrist from tenosynovitis of the surrounding tendons in the carpal tunnel. This causes a tingling sensation in the thumb, index and middle fingers of the affected hand and later weakness and wasting of the muscles at the base of the thumb. Symptoms are often worse in bed at night. Sometimes the condition can be helped by using a rest plaster on the wrist at night and may also be helped by injection of hydro-cortisone into the carpal tunnel. If these methods do not help then surgical decompression by cutting the compressing tissues overlying the nerve is simple and very effective. Other sites for compression of peripheral nerves are the ulnar nerve at the elbow and the lateral popliteal nerve at the knee.

Tendons, where surrounded by a synovial sheath, may become compressed if the sheath is inflamed. This inflammation may lead to the tendons becoming stuck within the sheaths, so reducing movement of the joint, and later may lead to rupture of the tendons. Tendons may also be ruptured where they lie close to bone which has become uneven because of arthritis. This acts like a saw as the tendons move across its surface. In the early stages where there is marked tenosynovitis removal of the inflamed synovium around affected tendons increases their range of movement and helps prevent rupture.

Tenotomy

The division of tendons (tenotomy) is occasionally needed when there is a severe contracture that has not responded to physical methods of treatment. This operation is sometimes combined with cutting the joint capsule which may also become contracted in long-standing deformity.

Synovectomy

At first sight this seems a very obvious and desirable operation. However, total removal of the synovium is usually not possible because of the complex shape of the joint cavities and sometimes there is very rapid regrowth of the synovium after operation. In addition, the immobilization that is needed post-operatively may leave the joint with some loss of movement and at times this may be considerable. The operation is usually carried out early in the course of the arthritis, after a period of conservative medical treatment with rest, splintage and local hydro-cortisone injections has failed. With the natural history of inflammatory arthritis improving of its own accord, accurate assessment of the results of synovectory can only be made by carrying out controlled trials. Two groups of patients, as near identical as possible, are treated by one group having synovectomy and the other being managed by non-surgical means and their joint status compared after an interval. Such trials are only just being carried out but it would seem that synovectomy of the knee and of the metacarpo-phalangeal joints in the hands is beneficial. Synovectomy of the proximal interphalangeal joints of the fingers is not of benefit. Synovectomy of the wrist, elbow and ankle has not yet been evaluated but is probably of benefit in certain cases. The difficulty is to know which cases will benefit.

> Joint Operations
>
> 1. Osteotomy
> 2. Arthrodesis
> 3. Arthroplasty

Joint Operations

We come now to the three major surgical operations carried out on joints, arthrodesis, osteotomy and arthroplasty. Five factors have to be considered in any operation on a joint: (1) relief of pain, (2) correction of any deformity, (3) the range of movement after operation, (4) stability of the joint after operation, and (5) the long-term effectiveness of the operation (see Fig. 16.1).

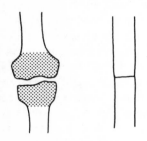

ARTHRODESIS

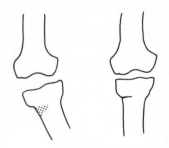

OSTEOTOMY

Arthrodesis		*Osteotomy*	
Relief of pain	Good	Relief of pain	Moderate to good
Correction of deformity	Good	Correction of deformity	Moderate
Range of movement	NIL	Range of movement	Moderate
Stability	Good	Stability	Moderate
Long-term effectiveness	Good	Long-term effectiveness	Moderate

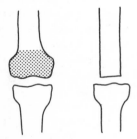

EXCISION ARTHROPLASTY

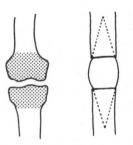

REPLACEMENT ARTHROPLASTY

Excision arthroplasty		*Replacement arthroplasty*
Relief of pain	Moderate to good	MCP joint with plastic insert
Correction of deformity	Moderate to good	The dotted lines represent
Range of movement	Moderate to excessive	intramedullary extensions
Stability	Very poor	of the arthroplasty. See
Long-term effectiveness	Moderate	p. 204, relief of pain, etc.

Fig. 16.1 Types of joint surgery. The pre–operative state is on the left and the shaded areas represent the bone removed at operation.

Arthrodesis

Arthrodesis means excision of the joint and bony fusion of the ends of the involved bones. If sound union of the bones follows there should be complete relief of pain; however, the emphasis must be on sound union as in arthritis very often the bones are osteoporotic and firm union after operation may not be complete. Deformity can be corrected. There is of course no movement possible after operation and this is the biggest disadvantage of the procedure. Although arthrodesis is in some respects a primitive procedure, it still has a place at certain joints. In the hands, arthrodesis of the proximal interphalangeal joints may be indicated if the fingers have already become fixed in either extension or gross flexion, provided that there is reasonable movement at the metacarpo-phalangeal joints. Arthrodesis of the wrists is still a very worthwhile operation. The loss of movement is not very restricting to the patient and again, provided sound union occurs, it allows the lifting and carrying of quite heavy objects without pain. The ankle cannot be regarded as a single joint, as the sub-taloid and mid-tarsal joints are also usually affected as well. Fusion of these three joints occasionally is indicated and again if union is sound, is very effective. Nowadays with the rapid advances that are occurring with arthroplasties, arthrodesis will gradually be replaced.

Osteotomy

Osteotomy means an operation in which one and sometimes both bones forming a joint are cut through and are then allowed to unite again. The process of cutting through the bones seems at times to reduce the pain from the joint although how this comes about is unknown. Although this used to be a common operation for arthritis of the hip, it has largely been replaced by arthroplasty. The only use now for osteotomy is when combined with correction of deformity at the joint by deliberate angulation of the divided bone. Used like this it is still occasionally a worthwhile procedure for knee joints, where it may improve flexion deformities and lateral deformities as well. Pain relief is usually not complete but is sufficient to satisfy most patients. The joint is fairly stable post-operatively. In ankylosing spondylitis osteotomy of the lumbar spine may be undertaken to improve posture if the spine is fixed in marked flexion, although it is an operation with considerable hazards because of possible damage to the spinal cord and its roots.

Arthroplasty

Arthroplasty means reconstruction of a joint. In its simplest form one or both bone ends of the affected joint are removed so that a gap is left. This is an excision arthroplasty, differing from osteotomy in that fusion of the bones is prevented. Excision arthroplasty results usually in considerable relief of pain and correction of deformity. The range of active movement is usually reduced and there is little

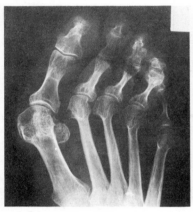 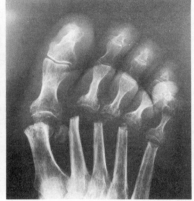

Fig. 16.2 X-ray of foot before Fowler's operation.

Fig. 16.3 X-ray of foot after Fowler's operation.

stability at the joint. The commonest site for this procedure is in the feet when there is subluxation of the metatarso-phalangeal joints. Here the heads of the metatarso-phalangeal bones are excised and this is known as Fowler's operation (Figs. 16.2 and 16.3). The result is usually very satisfactory with relief of pain and correction of the flexed toes. Usually patients find that they can wear normal shoes again and this is particularly important to women. Excision arthroplasty may also be effective at the wrist where excision of the lower end of an unstable ulna can produce great relief of pain. In the elbow excision of the head of the radius may improve pain particularly in pronation and supination movements.

Because of the instability that occurs this is not a suitable operation for larger joints that have to withstand considerable strain and attempts have therefore been made to replace the excised bone or bones by artificial means. At the present time this has only been predictably successful in one joint, the hip. Here at Wrightington

Hospital Sir John Charnley has successfully developed the use of a complete replacement for both elements in the hip joint. The artificial joint has a stainless steel femoral head and a high density plastic acetabular cup. Both components are fixed to bone by the use of a special bone cement which is not a glue but forms a perfect space-occupying material which moulds itself so tightly to its surroundings that it prevents movement. The results are usually complete relief of pain, correction of deformity, a very good range of movement and, after the first few weeks, good stability. In the long term there seems to be little wear of the artificial joint. However, the operation is a major one and the patients, who are often elderly, may have other illnesses such as diabetes, heart failure, etc. The hazards of the operation include deep vein thrombosis in the legs in the post-operative period with pulmonary embolus, and either immediate or late infection of the arthroplasty. Initially because of the uncertainties about how long the artificial joint would last the operation was restricted to people over the age of sixty-five; however, excessive wear has not proved to be a problem and this operation is now being carried out in younger people and particularly in younger rheumatoid patients where damage to other joints in the legs prevents them from putting excessive strain on the artificial joint. It is no exaggeration to say that this is an operation which has transformed the lives of thousands of people throughout the world.

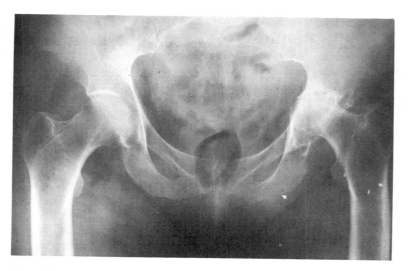

Fig. 16.4 X-ray of hips before operation. Note severe damage to left hip.

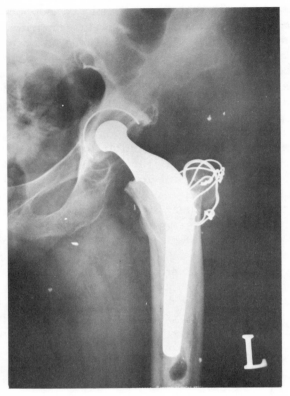

Fig. 16.5 X-ray of the hip after Charnley arthroplasty. The wires hold the greater trocanter in position until bony union occurs. The small white areas in the thigh are metal fragments from a war wound.

> Important Factors in Assessing Joint Surgery
>
> 1. Relief of pain
> 2. Correction of deformity
> 3. Stability of joint
> 4. Range of movement of joint
> 5. Long-term effectiveness

Attempts to achieve similar results at other joints have not been as successful and although replacement arthroplasty is available for the knee, metacarpo-phalangeal and elbow joints, its use at the moment must be regarded as very limited. But it would seem that over the next few years successful arthroplasties will be developed for these joints and probably eventually for virtually every peripheral joint in the body.

Further reading

Outline of Orthopaedics by J. Crawford Adams, (Churchill Livingstone).

17
Residual Disability

In this chapter we deal with the management of people who have some degree of permanent disability as a consequence of their arthritis. There is a tendency nowadays to say that if disability leads to a loss of function then the patient is handicapped. Inability to bend the fingers, for example, is a disability and the consequent inability to hold a cup represents a loss of function and handicap.

Particularly important at this stage of the patient's treatment are the occupational therapist, social worker and disablement resettlement officer. The work of these people will be described first and we will then discuss the management of permanent disability.

Occupational therapy

The work of the occupational therapist may be divided into three sections, assessment, therapy and diversion. In addition in some units the occupational therapist will be responsible for making splints and plasters.

ASSESSMENT. The type of assessment that is carried out will depend upon the type of illness being treated and we concentrate here upon the assessment of arthritic conditions. The initial emphasis in assessment is on those activities commonly called activities of daily living (ADL): eating, washing, dressing, toileting, housework, etc. There may, in addition, be assessment of particular problems at work or in travelling. Having assessed the problem the occupational therapist suggests either a different way of performing the task or the use of an aid to overcome the difficulty.

THERAPY. Here the object is to prescribe and supervise a series of 'occupations' (woodworking, weaving, etc) whose object is not to help pass the time for the patient but is aimed at improving muscle power, joint function and limb coordination. It may be considered, therefore, as a form of applied physiotherapy.

DIVERSION. Here the object is solely to occupy the patient's time. Occupational therapists should rarely be involved in this task, because of their high level of training and scarcity, although at times the edges between therapeutic and diversional regimes become very blurred.

We will now consider in more detail the work of the occupational therapist on a rheumatological unit under the first two headings of assessment and therapy.

Assessment. First a history of the patient's day is recorded and individual difficulties detailed. At times the occupational therapist may be able to predict that the patient will meet problems before the patient becomes aware of them himself. Following the history it is preferable to observe the patient in the difficult situations described by him. To allow for this, most occupational therapy departments have mock-ups of a kitchen, bathroom, bedroom and a living room. In these the patient's difficulties, for example, cooking a meal or getting in and out of a bath, can be observed. Some of the common problems in ADL are as follows.

DRESSING. The arthritic patient may, because of poor hand and arm function, have difficulty with fine finger movements for fastening buttons and pulling up zips, etc. Difficulty with buttons may be overcome by using a button hook or using 'false' buttons, where the button is sewn in place on the outside of the garment but closure is effected by velcro strips attached to the two surfaces to be joined and these are completely invisible when closed. Other common dressing problems for the arthritic are putting on stockings, fastening shoes and getting clothing around stiff shoulders (Figs. 17.1 to 17.4).

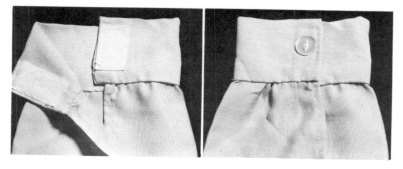

Fig. 17.1 Velcro used to make a false button fastening: (left) open, (right) closed.

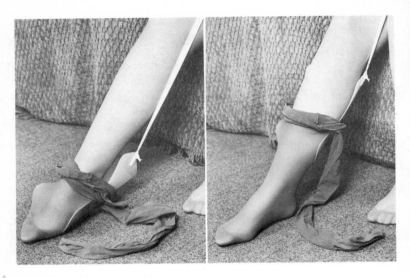

Fig. 17.2 Using a stocking gutter.

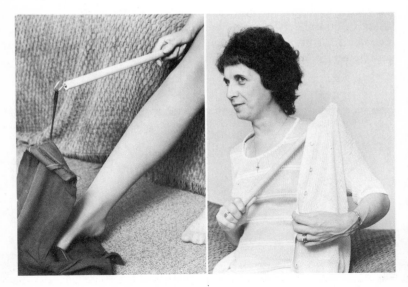

Fig. 17.3 Using a dressing stick.

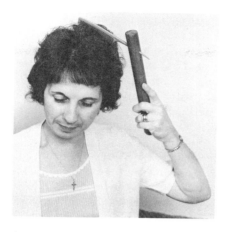

Fig. 17.4 Long-handled comb useful for someone with stiff shoulders.

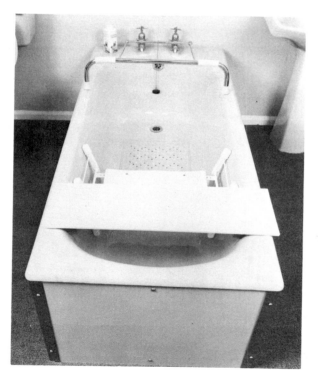

Fig. 17.5 Bath for a disabled person. Note bath board and seat, non-slip mat and grab rails around taps.

WASHING. Perhaps the commonest problem is difficulty getting into and out of the bath because of either painful knees or hips; upper limb disability may also contribute to the problems. A simple solution is the bath board (Fig. 17.5) and for the very disabled various types of hoists are available. An alternative solution may be to use a shower rather than a bath. Stiff or painful shoulders may make reaching to the back of the neck for washing impossible and the occupational therapist can usually provide an alternative way of doing this.

EATING. Arthritis affecting the hands may make it difficult to use the standard knife and fork and this may occur quite early in the disease. The easy answer is to thicken the handles of knives and forks with either plastic or wood (Fig. 17.6). Later, with severe deformity of the hands more individual adaptations may be needed (Fig. 17.7).

TOILETING. A very common problem with limited hip movements and/or painful knees is difficulty in sitting on a toilet of normal

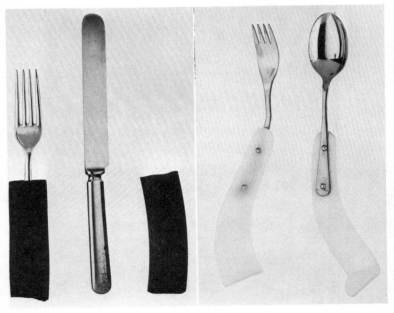

Fig. 17.6 Simple thickening of handles of knife and fork.

Fig. 17.7 More complicated alterations to handles of cutlery.

height. The answer is usually to raise the toilet seat, either permanently or temporarily and to surround the toilet with grab rails at the correct sites.

KITCHEN. In the kitchen many difficulties may be encountered including lifting heavy pans full of hot fat or boiling water or reaching up to high shelving. Women patients are usually asked to cook a meal in

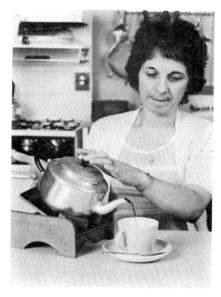

Fig. 17.8 Tilting teapot stand.

the occupational therapy kitchen when any problems rapidly become apparent and the patient can be shown alternative techniques to use.

In general an aid should be (1) simple in design
(2) acceptable to the patient
(3) as 'normal' in appearance as possible
(4) as cheap as possible
(5) as long lasting as possible
(6) capable of being altered if the patient's disability alters

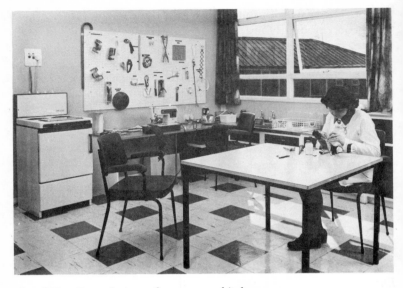

Fig. 17.9   General view of assessment kitchen.

Therapy. This needs further space in the occupational therapy department to provide facilities for woodworking, weaving, light and heavy mechanical workshops. With these available occupational therapy can be arranged for all varieties of disability. This therapy encourages the patient to concentrate on what he can do rather than on the negative attitude of what he cannot do. The patient's ability to concentrate and his endurance can be observed and increased. As a consequence useful advice about employment can often be given.

Social worker

A social worker may find himself involved in many aspects of an arthritic patient's illness. He may indeed be involved with a patient before he is admitted to hospital, perhaps because an aged relative will have to be found temporary alternative accommodation and on occasions elderly spinsters have been known to need their pets boarding out before they can be admitted! After admission the social worker takes a history from the patient, paying particular attention to details about the family, the number of children, type of housing and, if possible, the financial situation. Other likely problem areas such as work and travel will be discussed with the patient. He may visit the family at home and talk, with the patient's permission, to the patient's employer. He will attempt to define those areas of stress in the life of the patient and his family that are causing most concern.

He is responsible for seeing that the patient receives all the benefits that the government has made available for chronically disabled people. The patient may be entitled to financial help from a constant attendance allowance, mobility allowance or supplementary benefit. The social worker helps the patient make these claims.

Working with a disablement resettlement officer (DRO) he helps the patient find, if possible, suitable employment. Help may be needed either to re-house the patient, usually to single storey accommodation or to adapt the present home by providing ramps for outdoor steps and other alterations. The social worker liaises with his colleagues in the community over these changes. When the patient is discharged contact may be passed to the care of a community social worker.

Disablement resettlement officer (DRO)

The DRO is especially trained to assess and advise disabled people about the possibility of returning to work. He may recommend that the patient becomes a registered disabled person. This may increase his chances of being employed, as by law all firms employing more than 20 people have to employ a 'quota' of registered disabled people. He may recommend that a period of more detailed assessment, followed by re-training at what used to be called an Industrial Rehabilitation Unit (IRU) but is now known as an Employment Resettlement Centre (ERC) would be best for the patient.

Residual disability

We have now seen the large number of people who may take part in the treatment of an arthritic patient: rheumatologist, surgeon, nurse, physiotherapist, occupational therapist, social worker and disablement resettlement officer. If this large number of people are to work together there must be coordination and understanding of what is being attempted and everyone must work together as a team. Each member of the team must be an expert in his own field and must also have an appreciation of, and respect for, the work of the other members of the team. Such teams take time to become established but an established team has an easy confidence in what it can and should do and this conficence is rapidly transmitted to the patient.

The nursing members of the team must therefore be not only competent as nurses but must understand the work of the other team members. They should be able to explain to their patient the functions of the para-medical staff and be familiar with the techniques that they employ. They must be aware of the impact of chronic disease not only on the patient but also on relatives. They will be aware of situations when extra anxiety may be expected, for example, while waiting for surgery. They will try always to look for those personal qualities that differentiate one patient from another.

There is often a difference between what can be done for the patient and what should be done. It is possible to indulge in sophisticated surgery to replace a hip joint, only to find that when the patient returns home he resumes his seat beside the fire and rarely leaves it. What has been gained? The multiple observations of the patient by the team members should prevent this sort of situation occurring and should permit the setting up of more realistic targets. With very complex physical problems there are often special problems and a 'case conference' is often the best way to sort out a realistic target in this situation. Present at the conference, called after the patient has been in hospital for at least a few days assessment, will be as many members of the team as possible, plus the patient and his relatives. We have now introduced the last and most important members of the team, the patient and his family. We must not think of the arthritic patient in isolation but should always remember that he is usually part of a family.

Arthritis may be a long illness and may lead to serious disability and this may have drastic effects on the other members of the family. If it is the man who is affected he may have to change work and usually earn less money as a consequence. If more severely affected he may be unable to work at all and sometimes then the wife goes out to work and the husband stays at home and looks after the house. The man may find this 'role reversal' situation difficult to accept. He may feel that his position as wage-earner and head of the household has been lost and may suffer great loss of confidence in himself as a consequence.

If it is the woman who is affected by arthritis she will almost certainly not be able to cope with looking after several children, the housework and shopping. The husband has to take over some of these duties and these have to be done when he returns from work. It is not difficult to imagine the strain of returning from work to a home which needs cleaning and having to prepare the evening meal.

Whether it be the man or woman who is affected it will be seen that the marriage will be put under considerable strain.

Sexual problems

Sexual difficulties are common. A survey has shown that at least 50% of arthritic patients find that the arthritis has interfered with their sexual lives and 25% stated that this was causing marital stress. Depression and loss of libido may reduce the desire for intercourse, pain and stiffness in joints may make it too painful. There is probably a higher than average divorce and separation rate in arthritic families. At the moment it is difficult for these patients to get advice about their problems but the Arthritis and Rheumatism Council have produced a free handbook, Marriage, Sex and Arthritis. It is our policy to give this to all patients admitted to our unit. Besides providing information for the patient, it indicates that we are prepared to discuss this aspect of arthritis. If problems are raised, combined interviews with the patient and spouse are essential. Frequently all that is required is an explanation to the non-affected partner of how the arthritis is affecting the patient's sexual life and advice about differing positions being used for intercourse. The doctor's role is often to re-assure couples that these variations are permissible and are in no way perverted.

Pregnancy

Pregnancy is not contra-indicated in most forms of arthritis, although in SLE with renal damage this may be made worse. Ideally, pregnancy should be planned so that conception occurs when the disease is in a remission and most of the drug therapy has been discontinued, to prevent any hazard to the fetus. Steroids usually need to be continued but do not seem a danger to the fetus. The joint status should be assessed before conception, bearing in mind that the hips and knees will carry extra strain during pregnancy and that hands and wrist joints will be strained looking after the newborn child. It might therefore be advisable in some cases to consider surgery before the patient becomes pregnant. Rheumatoid arthritis usually improves during the course of pregnancy, perhaps due to metabolic changes associated with pregnancy. After delivery there is likely to be a flare up of the arthritis and this may be made worse by the increase in physical activity in looking after the child. Some drugs are excreted in the mother's milk and this needs to be borne in mind if

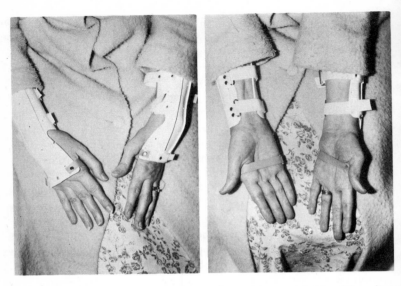

Fig. 17.10 Special wrist splints for mothers with young babies. The splints support the wrist in extension but leave the palm free for safe lifting.

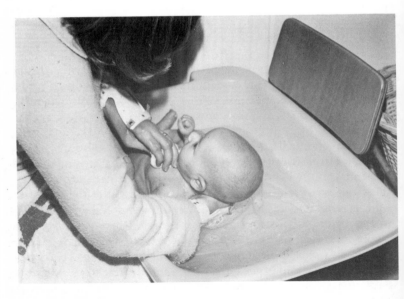

Fig. 17.11 Splints in use.

the mother intends to breast feed. As we have stated before this is not the time to separate mother and child and if the mother's condition deteriorates enough to warrant hospital admission, it is our policy to admit both mother and child to a side ward. Here the mother can feed, wash and dress the baby, while relieved of all household chores. Sometimes special wrist splints are needed to allow the mother with painful wrists to lift the baby with confidence (Figs. 17.10 and 17.11).

Problems of arthritic children

Children with arthritis have special problems. In children, as in adults, arthritis may range from a relatively minor illness, affecting only one or two joints, to a protracted illness lasting many years and affecting many joints. With severe polyarthritis, some degree of failure to grow to a normal height is common. This follows as a consequence of the disease and may be made worse by steroid treatment which also reduces growth. There may be premature fusion of the epiphyses around an inflamed joint resulting in a limb that is shorter than the non-affected side. In both sexes puberty may be delayed.

With severe disease, prolonged periods of hospitalization may be needed and even mild disease will probably need one or two short periods of hospital admission. Prolonged hospitalization in a child has special problems. Separation from the other members of the family and lack of stimulus from day to day events which occur at home, leave the child isolated. Schooling may be lost. Continuing education is probably as important as medical treatment for the arthritis. The child with arthritis, when he becomes an adult, will probably not be able to earn a living in a manual occupation and has to work using his brains rather than his joints. As an adult he is likely to be at a physical disadvantage compared to his friends and must not be allowed to become inferior in education as well. This means that if a child with arthritis needs to be hospitalized for any length of time, schooling must be continued and be regarded as part of the day's routine treatment. If possible, regular visits from the ward to places of interest, such as zoos, should be encouraged.

Emotional problems are common. A child's frustration at not being able to take part in the activities of his friends may be converted to anger which is vented on his parents and siblings. Parents have continually to be on the look-out to avoid over-protecting the child and yielding to his every demand simply because he is ill.

Brothers and sisters are likely to be jealous of the disproportionate amount of parental time spent on the arthritic child.

As puberty approaches sexual problems may develop. Girls with severe deformities of the hands may find coping with menstruation difficult and may need the help of an occupational therapist. Both sexes may have delayed puberty and will worry about this. It needs to be explained to them that eventually they will develop sexually. Girls need reassurance that they will be able to have children and that

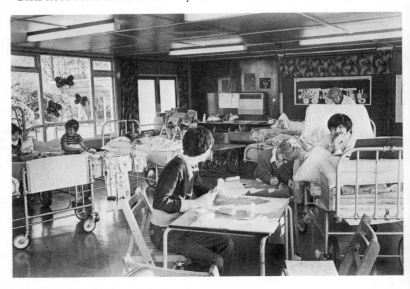

Fig. 17.12   The hospital school.

the chance of these children having arthritis is very small. Boys by being over-protected, may have difficulties in developing these qualities which society regards as masculine. Both sexes, because of their restricted mobility, may find difficulty in making friends.

The arthritic family

If the arthritic family are to gain the maximum support from the hospital service they must be fully aware of the diagnosis and of any complications that are present. They should understand what treatment is being used and the objects of that treatment. They should be familiar with the names of the drugs being taken and of their more important side effects. Some idea of the prognosis should have been given. They should have found that the team are interested in them as a family unit and feel that they can turn to the team for help in matters which may not seem to them strictly medical. In order to help in educating patients the Arthritis and Rheumatism Council have produced a series of free booklets on various types of arthritis and these should be available for the patient and his relatives.

Disability and society

Education needs to extend further than the patient and his family; it needs to extend into society in general. It is society which decides which loss of function is going to be a handicap. Short- or long-sightedness is a loss of function but is not a handicap as glasses are freely available. Compare this with the lack of provision for people in wheelchairs: difficulty with crossing the road due to high kerbs, difficulty with entering buildings because of high steps, etc. A wheelchair life is a severe handicap; but it is we who have created this difficulty by not ensuring that solutions to these problems are available. In a suitable environment, and several villages exist in Europe which have been designed from the start with these problems in mind, the normal population and the disabled can live side by side with almost equal mobility.

Rehabilitation

Some people would apply this word to much of the work described above. In general we disapprove of the idea that rehabilitation is a special type of treatment that can only be carried out in a separate establishment. In our view, with one or two exceptions, there is no time at which medical treatment can be said to have ended and rehabilitation started. Indeed, it can be said that rehabilitation starts in the ambulance on the way to hospital. We hope in the future that those aspects of treatment that are now called rehabilitation will increasingly be carried out by the physician or surgeon in charge of the acute illness.

Further reading

Coping with disablement. Consumers Association.
Sex and the physically handicapped. National Fund for Research into Crippling Diseases.
Rheumatoid Arthritis. ARC handbook.
Marriage, Sex and Arthritis. ARC handbook.
Dressing for disabled people. R. Rushton. Disabled Living Foundation.
Other ARC handbooks.

Appendix A
Home Exercises for
Ankylosing Spondylitis

Breathing Exercises

1   Lie flat on your back on a firm bed. Place your hands on the
     sides of your chest over the lower ribs, then breathe slowly in
     and out feeling the amount of movement under your hands.

Head and Neck

1   Bend your head forwards and backwards as far as possible,
     especially backwards.
2   Keeping your head upright, turn it from side to side as far as
     possible.
3   Facing forwards, bend your head to left and right.

Hips and Knees

Lie flat on bed or on floor

1   Bend your right knee, then straighten knee and lower leg to the
     bed, keeping your knee straight; repeat with left leg.
2   Separate your feet as far as you can and then bring your feet
     together again.

Back

1   Bend your knees and place your feet firmly on the floor. Now
     lift your hips off the floor and get as straight a line from your
     knees to your shoulders as possible.
2   Keeping your knees bent and keeping your knees together and
     your shoulders on the bed, now roll your knees first to the left
     and then to the right.
3   Lie on your front with your hands by your sides. Now try to
     lift your head and shoulders off the floor.
     Try and spend some time each day lying flat on your front with
     your head turned to one side.
     Standing as straight as possible, lift your hands over your head.
     Now bend forward and try to touch your toes.

Shoulders

1   Bend your elbows and place your fingers on the tips of your
     shoulders. Now take your arms around in as large a circle as
     possible.

Appendix B
Questions Patients
Ask about Arthritis

It is our policy to have informal meetings with the ward patients. These are usually held in the day room and are attended by all the patients and one consultant and the ward sister. We recognize that the formal ward round with up to ten people assembled around the patient can be very inhibiting for the patient. The situation in the day room meeting is reversed and we are outnumbered at least ten to one. This encourages patients to ask questions and we list below the commoner questions asked and you may be sure that if you work with arthritics you will be asked most of these questions by your patients. If you have read the book so far you should be able to answer these questions without further help. However, just to make sure we provide over the page our answers and comments.

1 Does the arthritis ever burn itself out?
2 Why does it flare up?
3 Does stress cause arthritis?
4 Is rheumatoid arthritis hereditary?
5 Is there a set amount of gold to have?
6 Everybody says keep going but when you come into hospital you are told to rest. Which is correct?
7 Why does gold not suit everybody?
8 Why don't they tell you the side effects of drugs?
9 What is the safe dose of steroids?
10 Are you more liable to infection with steroids?
11 Are heat lamps any good?
12 Should I have out-patient physiotherapy after discharge?
13 What is the difference between rheumatoid arthritis and osteoarthrosis?
14 What is the relationship between psoriasis and joint disease?
15 Do you think that diet can play a part in the treatment of arthritis?
16 Is acupuncture of any benefit for arthritics?
17 Does the weather affect joint symptoms?
18 Why does my face swell so badly when I take cortisone when it does not seem to affect other people?
19 Could you tell me why my shoulders and hands seem to have grown worse and more painful since doing the exercises?

20 May the eyesight be affected in any way in arthritis?
21 Is alcohol allowed in arthritis?

Answers
(1) Does the arthritis ever burn itself out?
Answer: Yes, but it may take some years to do so.
Comment: Although this may not be strictly true, we feel it is
important to hold out some ray of hope to patients with
inflammatory arthritis.

(2) Why does it flare up?
Answer: Inflammatory arthritis may flare up from overuse of
the joints, failure to take tablets, and may be worse if some
intercurrent infection, such as tonsillitis, occurs.
Comment: Ask the patient what condition makes his arthritis
flare up. Use this to emphasize the benefit of rest in inflamed
joints.

(3) Does stress cause arthritis?
Answer: Both rheumatoid arthritis and stress are very common.
Therefore, not uncommonly the two will occur together. It is
our belief that stress does not cause rheumatoid arthritis,
although it may make the symptoms worse.
Comment: Give as an example how when you have a cold
everything seems that much more difficult to do.

(4) Is rheumatoid arthritis hereditary?
Answer: There is a slightly increased incidence of rheumatoid
arthritis in people who are close relatives of a patient with
rheumatoid arthritis. However, rheumatoid arthritis is very
common and because of this, occasional groupings of patients
are bound to occur and it is in these sorts of cases that there is a
very strong family history.

(5) Is there a set amount of gold to have?
Answer: No. Gold is given until either there is a response, when
it is reduced to a maintenance dosage or when it is seen not to be
effective, which usually means after twenty injections.

(6) Everybody says keep going, but when you come into hospital you are told to rest. Which is correct?
Answer: Most people are afraid that they will stiffen up if they
rest their joints. This is because they feel so stiff first thing in the

morning and the stiffness improves later in the day. Nevertheless, using painful joints in inflammatory arthritis makes them
worse.

Comment: Most patients after resting for a few days in bed in
hospital feel very much better and this can be pointed out to
them at the time. Again this is a teaching situation where
emphasis can be given on resting acutely painful joints.

(7) Why does gold not suit everybody?
Answer: We do not know. Most drugs suit some people and not
others.

(8) Why don't they tell you the side effects of drugs?
Answer: It is our policy to tell you the main side effects and in
particular those which may be dangerous. However, we do not
like to over-emphasize the side effects from drugs.
Comment: Point out to the patient that in controlled trials there
are frequently as many reactions amongst people who are taking
placebo tablets as amongst those taking the actual drug being
tested.

(9) What is a safe dose of steroids?
Answer: It is usually recognized that a dose of 7.5 mg of prednisolone a day is the maximum long-term maintenance dose
which produces the maximum improvement with the
minimum of side effects.

(10) Are you more liable to infection with steroids?
Answer: Yes, and it is important that you let any doctor know
that you are on steroids if you become ill. It is also important
that you do not stop taking your steroids if you become ill and
sometimes indeed you need to have an increased dose of steroids
if you have another illness. You should carry your steroid card
with you at all times.

(11) Are heat lamps any good?
Answer: Heat is very comforting to inflamed joints. We use it in
hospital before carrying out certain exercises. Any form of heat
is suitable and hot water is the best for hands, for example, and a
hot water bottle is cheaper than any form of lamp.

(12) Should I have out-patient physiotherapy after discharge?
Answer: It is usually not necessary to have physiotherapy after
discharge. You should continue to do the daily exercises which
you have been shown how to do in here.

Comment: It is important not to encourage people to attend physiotherapy departments on an occasional basis because they feel it does them good. Physiotherapy, if needed, should be an intensive form of treatment.

(13) What is the difference between rheumatoid arthritis and osteoarthrosis?

Answer: This is one of the most difficult questions to answer; it is difficult to explain the difference to nurses and even to some doctors. Rheumatoid arthritis is an inflammation of the joints whereas in osteoarthrosis, there is degeneration of the joints. There is little or no inflammation in the joints in osteoarthrosis, and no prolonged stiffness of the joints in the morning. Treatment of the two conditions is very different.

Comment: Emphasize this difference and in particular point out that systemic steroids have no effect in osteoarthrosis.

(14) What is the relationship between psoriasis and joint disease?

Answer: Some patients with psoriasis develop arthritis and this arthritis may be different from rheumatoid arthritis and is called psoriatic arthritis. Treatment is similar to rheumatoid arthritis but in general the outlook is much better than in rheumatoid arthritis.

(15) Do you think that diet can play a part in the treatment of arthritis?

Answer: You can have an entirely normal diet. The only thing to watch is your weight. You must not become overweight. Otherwise you can eat whatever you want.

Comment: Emphasize to patients that they can eat acid foods, whatever these may be, as patients often believe that acid is the cause of arthritis.

(16) Is acupuncture of any benefit?

Answer: It may provide some short-term relief of pain.

Comment: Ask the patient if he felt any benefit. If he did then explain that acupuncture certainly cannot do any harm but do not encourage him to spend large amounts of money on this treatment.

(17) Does the weather affect joint symptoms?

Comment: In a group discussion ask how many patients feel better in hot weather and how many feel better in cold weather. You will usually find that the group is split 50–50.

(18) Why does my face swell so badly when I take cortisone when it does not seem to affect other people?

Answer: Partly this depends upon the amount of cortisone you take. If you are on too high a dose your face certainly will swell. Nevertheless, cortisone does seem to affect people differently and some people do show this swelling of the face more than other people.

Comment: Again emphasize to the patient the importance of not stopping the steroids and not changing the dosage himself.

(19) Could you tell me why my shoulders and hands seem to have grown worse and more painful since doing the exercises?

Comment: We seem to have slipped up here and given the patient more exercise than his joints can currently stand. Therefore, explain again that over-usage of the joints makes them worse. Emphasize to the patient that it is important that he tells us if he has any fresh symptoms after admission and in particular how they are responding to treatment.

(20) May the eyesight be affected in any way in arthritis?

Answer: Yes. Depending on the type of arthritis there may be various eye complications.

Comment: Remember that iritis occurs with the sero-negative group of arthritides, that Sjögren's syndrome produces dry eyes, and that conjunctivitis is an early symptom of Reiter's disease. In children, particularly those with only one or two joints involved and the presence of a positive ANF test, iritis is not uncommon.

(21) Is alcohol allowed in arthritis?

Answer: Yes.

Comment: All is not black in arthritis!

Appendix C
Useful addresses

Arthritis and Rheumatism Council	8–10 Charing Cross Road, London WC2H OHN
Back Pain Association	Grundy House, Somerset Road, Teddington, Middlesex TW1 8RD

British Association for Rheumatology and Rehabilitation	Royal College of Physicians, 11 St. Andrews Place, Regent's Park, London NW1 4LE
British Council for Rehabilitation of the Disabled	Tavistock House, Tavistock Square, London WC1H 9LB
British League against Rheumatism	8 Charing Cross Road, London WC2H 0HN
British Rheumatism and Arthritis Association	1 Devonshire Place, London W1N 2BD
British Sports Association for the Disabled	Stoke Mandeville Stadium, Harvey Road, Aylesbury, Buckinghamshire
Central Council for the Disabled	34 Eccleston Square, London SW1N IPE
Consumers Association	14 Buckingham Street, London WC2
Disabled Living Foundation	346 Kensington High Street, London W14
Disabled Alliance	96 Portland Place, London W1
Psoriasis Association	7 Milton Street, Northampton NN2 7JG
Rehabilitiation Engineering Movement Advisory Panels (REMAP)	Thames House North, Millbank, London SW1P 4QG
Scottish Committee for the Welfare of the Disabled.	19 Claremont Crescent, Edinburgh EH7 4QD
Sexual Problems of the Disabled (SPOD)	Vincent House, 1 Springfield Road, Horsham, Sussex
Wales Council for the Disabled	2 Cathedral Road, Cardiff
Wrightington Hospital	Wigan, Lancashire

Glossary of Terms and Abbreviations

Arthritis: is used to describe inflammation of a joint. In the past it was used to describe all types of joint disease

Arthritides: plural of arthritis

Arthropathy: a disease of joints

Arthrosis: a non-inflammatory disease of joints, ie osteoarthrosis

Arteritis: inflammation of an artery

Ankylosis: the replacement of a joint by bone (bony ankylosis) or by fibrous tissue (fibrous ankylosis)

Arthralgia: pain in joints with no abnormality on clinical examination

Arthrodesis: surgical removal of a joint with fusion of the bones

Arthrogram: the radiographic appearances of a joint after a radio-opaque substance has been injected into the bone cavity

Arthroplasty: surgical reconstruction of a joint

Arthroscopy: a technique to allow inspection of the interior of a joint through a special instrument

Biopsy: removal of tissue (synovium, bone, etc) to help in the diagnosis

Electromyography: records the electrical activity occurring in muscles and nerves. Useful in the diagnosis of muscle and nerve disease

Erosions: the punched out lesions in bone seen on radiographs. Typically present in rheumatoid arthritis, but seen also in many other types of joint disease

Goniometer: an instrument used to measure the range of joint movement

Haemarthrosis: the presence of blood in the joint cavity

Kyphosis: an excessive posterior curvature of the spine (convex posteriorly)

Lordosis: the opposite of kyphosis

Mono-neuritis multiplex: paralysis of a peripheral nerve often due to arteritis of the artery supplying the nerve. Called multiplex as several peripheral nerves may be affected at the same time.

Myalgia: pain in the muscles

Myopathy: a word used to cover all disease of muscle, ie inflammatory myopathy, metabolic myopathy, etc

Myositis: inflammation of muscles. May occur by itself as in polymyositis or with skin lesions as in dermatomyositis. Myositis also occurs in rheumatoid arthritis and other connective tissue diseases

Myelogram: the introduction of radio-opaque material into the cerebro-spinal fluid in order to outline the nerves and spinal cord within the spinal canal.

Nodules: sub-cutaneous 'lumps' which may be seen in rheumatoid arthritis. A different type is seen in rheumatic fever

Osteomyelitis: infection of bone

Osteophyte: a bony outgrowth that occurs at the joint margin in osteoarthrosis

Osteotomy: an operation in which one or both bones forming the joint are cut through and then allowed to re-unite

Pannus: inflamed synovial tissue which erodes cartilage and bone

Periostium: the thin layer of tissue that surrounds the shafts of bones

Prosthesis: an artificial replacement for a human part, ie artificial leg, artificial hip joint, etc

Rheumatism: pain arising from muscles, tendons or joints

Scoliosis: a lateral bending of the spine

Spondylitis: inflammation of the spinal joints

Spondylosis: multiple degenerative changes of vertebral discs with osteophyte formation; OA of the spine

Synovectomy: surgical removal of synovium

Synovium: thin layer of tissue lining the joint capsule which produces synovial fluid

Synovitis: inflammation of synovium

Tendonitis: inflammation of a tendon

Tenosynovitis: inflammation of the synovial sheath surrounding tendons

Tenotomy: cutting a tendon, commonly in such a fashion as to lengthen the tendon

Vasculitis: inflammation of blood vessels

Xerostomia: a dry mouth

ANA antinuclear antibody
ANF antinuclear factor (identical to ANA)
AS ankylosing spondylitis
ASA acetylsalicylic acid (aspirin)
ASOT anti-streptolysin titre
CPP calcium pyrophosphate
DRO Disablement Resettlement Officer

EMG electromyography
ESR erythrocyte sedimentation rate
GOA generalized osteoarthrosis
HLA human leucocyte antigen
JCA juvenile chronic arthritis
JRA juvenile rheumatoid arthritis
LE cell lupus erythematosus cell
MCC metacarpal carpal joint
MCP metacarpal phalangeal joint
MTP metatarsal phalangeal joint
OA osteoarthrosis
PID prolapsed intervertebral disc
PIP proximal interphalangeal joint
POP plaster of Paris
RA rheumatoid arthritis
SCAT sheep cell agglutination test
SIJ sacroiliac joint
SLE systemic lupus erythematosus
TIP terminal interphalangeal joint

Index